Welfare Medical Care

Welfare Medical Care

An experiment

Charles H. Goodrich, M.D.
Margaret C. Olendzki, Ph.D.
George G. Reader, M.D.

Harvard University Press
Cambridge, Massachusetts
1970

Distributed in Great Britain by Oxford University Press, London

SBN 674-94895-5
Library of Congress Catalog Card Number 77-85075
Printed in the United States of America

Preface

The New York Hospital–Cornell Project, 1960–1965, was an experiment in the organization of welfare medical care services. It evolved in response to the concern of the New York City Departments of Health and Welfare with the quality and cost of medical care available to welfare clients. Building on long research experience within the Comprehensive Care and Teaching Program, the New York Hospital Cornell Medical Center undertook an experimental program of care for welfare families.

Determining the feasibility of such an undertaking was the demonstration aspect of the Project. This part will be presented as a description of what happened at the New York Hospital with the patients who came for care. The Project, however, was also a controlled experiment designed to compare two systems of medical care: the existing system and the experimental system within which the demonstration took place. Therefore, subjects for the study group were randomly selected from new admissions to welfare in the local districts and invited to obtain all their medical care from the New York Hospital. At the same time, a control group was similarly selected and left to obtain their care under the existing arrangements; and the two systems of care were compared along the dimensions of utilization, cost, and quality of care, including patient satisfaction.

The genesis of the Project and the characteristics of the welfare population who served as subjects for the study are reported on in Part I. In Part II, the experience of staff and patients at the New York Hospital is described and analyzed. In Part III, the focus of attention is moved from one medical institution to the whole city, and the total study group system of care (including those of the study group who never came to the New York Hospital) is compared with the existing system of medical care represented by the control group. The findings presented in the report are summarized and commented upon in the concluding chapter.

The question of the feasibility of such a complete-care program had several aspects. To begin with, enough patients had to be persuaded to use the designated facility for their medical care, rather than those facilities to which they were perhaps more accustomed. Despite the fact that the New York Hospital was further than other hospitals from the homes of many of the welfare clients and that it was unfamiliar to most of them, a large number of patients were persuaded to turn to the New York Hospital as their main source of medical care.

Other aspects of feasibility involved the institution offering care. The provision of complete medical care to a section of a community constitutes a departure from ordinary practice for most hospitals and had to be planned to avoid disrupting the other missions of a university hospital. Education and research are important functions for a teaching hospital, and service obligations should be coordinated with these goals if such an institution is to accomplish its purpose. Routine service responsibilities should not impair the ability of the teaching hospital to serve as a referral center for complicated clinical problems. And the expense of service to the indigent should not be borne by a voluntary hospital if public funds are available for welfare medical care. These problems were resolved in the Project by careful planning of the size of the demonstration and its relationship to the regular facilities and ancillary services of the New York Hospital. Special clinical and administrative staff, whose job was to coordinate the Project with the usual functions of the hospital, had to be recruited. Most of the expenses for medical services in the demonstration were met through a pre-payment contract with the Welfare Department and from grant funds, although a significant contribution was still needed from the hospital because of inadequacies of the reimbursement mechanism.

A major research challenge was to secure comparable data on study and control groups for the comparison of the two systems of medical care. Adequate records were hard to find or unavailable in many instances from providers of service other than the New York Hospital. But the household interviews conducted by the National Opinion Research Center provided more complete and accurate information on sources and volume of medical services than had been anticipated. It was therefore possible to obtain useful data from which significant comparisons could be made between the two alternative systems of care.

The New York Hospital–Cornell Welfare Medical Care Project was generously supported by a five-year research grant from the Health Research Council (contract U-1042). Preparation of this report was facilitated by a one year Health Research Council grant (contract U-1667), by support of the Research Administration Committee of Mount Sinai School of Medicine (Fund 74-2005), by a Program Grant in Patient Care Research from the United States Public Health Service (CH 00103), and by the Commonwealth Fund of New York. In addition, the Health Economics Branch of the United States Public Health Service provided consultation and financial assistance in the interpretation of some of the data.

The Project had its immediate origin in a task force, chaired by Dr. George James, which met first in 1959 to consider ways of improving welfare medical care. Dr. George Baehr, as a member of the task force, made the recommendation for a coordinated-care experiment based in a voluntary hospital. The city then turned to Cornell University and the New York Hospital for implementation of the recommendation. For the city, Dr. Leona Baumgartner, commissioner of health, and Mr. James Dumpson, commissioner of welfare, helped formulate the Project; and Dr. E. Hugh Luckey, physician-in-chief of the New York Hospital, Dr. Henry Pratt, director of the New York Hospital, and Dr. John Deitrick, dean of the Cornell Medical College, acted for the Center. Dr. Charles Goodrich and Dr. Margaret Olendzki assumed the responsibility for planning and organizing the Project under the supervision of Dr. George Reader, professor of Medicine, Cornell Medical College, as principal investigator.

Special thanks are due the city Departments of Health and Welfare and particularly Dr. George James, then first deputy commissioner of health, Dr. Paul Densen, then deputy commissioner of health for research, and Dr. Alonzo Yerby, then director of welfare medical care, for their guidance in carrying out a project that was in many ways a collaborative endeavor. Mr. Jerome Cornfield, then of the United States Public Health Service, gave valuable advice and help in his role of statistical consultant.

Many others helped at crucial points in the study. Indeed, it could not have been brought to successful completion without the unstinting cooperation provided by the staffs of the Departments of Health and Welfare and of the medical center. Mr. Henry Rosner and Mr. Michael Rappaport of the Department of Welfare deserve mention, as do Mr. John Keig, comptroller of the New York Hospital, and Mrs. Treherne-Thomas, director of volunteers. Dr. Mary E. W. Goss, associate professor of sociology in medicine, Cornell Medical College, served as a valuable consultant throughout the course of the study.

Mr. Paul Sheatsley of the National Opinion Research Center and Mr. Donald Kabat of Arthur Andersen & Co. made the resources of their organizations readily available to the investigators.

From its outset, the Project was conceived as a clinical investigation of welfare medical care. Both the medical care plan and the research design were shaped and carried out by clinicians and social scientists. In the truest sense, this final report is the product of a team effort. For this reason, the editors have not identified the individual contributions of each member of the team. Instead, we have listed those who participated in the actual writing of the report as associate editors or contributors. Every member of the Project staff, however, played an important part in the rendering of care or the collection and analysis of data.

Mr. David Ilk deserves special mention for his volunteer work throughout the Project, which provided consistent, accurate recording of utilization data from the hospital charts. We are also grateful to Mrs. Marion Goodrich for her help in typing and editing the many drafts of the manuscript; to Mr. Nicholas Childs for his meticulous checking of the statistical data; and to Mrs. Lucille Goodlet for her careful review of every aspect of the report through all stages of its preparation.

C. G.

M. O.

G. G. R.

Contents

Tables

Appendix A: Supplementary Tables (A-1 to A-43)

Figures

One | Background and Development

1 | The Development of the New York Hospital — Cornell Project

The purpose of the New York Hospital–Cornell Welfare Medical Care Project was to determine whether or not it was feasible for a voluntary teaching hospital to provide complete medical care to a population of welfare recipients and to study the utilization, cost, and quality of this care.

For many years the Health and Welfare Departments of the City of New York have been interested in improving the quality of medical care for the welfare client. The interest of the Welfare Department in the health of its clients, as well as in their general support, can be traced back to 1867, when the Board of State Commissioners of Public Charities was given responsibility for supervision of all charitable institutions. Hospitals at that time were defined as charitable institutions, as they still are today, and therefore fell under the aegis of a welfare agency. When a city Public Health Board was established, it was mainly concerned with environmental health problems such as sanitation, water supply, and the control of epidemics. But it did later establish sanatoria for the tuberculous and special diagnostic and treatment centers for venereal diseases. Its citywide health centers also served the health needs of the indigent population, especially the children. Thus, through much of their history, health and welfare departments tended to work in different areas of health rather than in close collaboration.

Recently, however, the need for such collaboration has been fully realized. This was clearly expressed as a challenge by Leona Baumgartner and James Dumpson in their article, "Health in Welfare: A Joint or a Divided Responsibility".[1] Under their leadership, New York City entered a period of experimentation with various methods of improving the care of the indigent. The Health Department, because of its increasing preoccupation with the primary health problem of the community, chronic illness, was finding its way into the business of medical care. The Welfare Department, in its traditional role of financial contributor to the costs of indigent medical care, needed the assistance and professional leadership of the Health Department to raise the quality of medical care.

The New York Hospital–Cornell Medical Center, which was founded in 1771 as a voluntary hospital and was affiliated in 1927 with Cornell University Medical College, has traditionally been interested both in improving the coordination of care within the hospital and in extending its services into the community; it also has a tradition of patient-care research and experimentation. In the 1920's the Cornell Pay Clinic

---

1. Leona Baumgartner and James R. Dumpson, *American Journal of Public Health,* 52:1067-1076 (July 1962).

experimented with the organization of medical services by endeavoring to offer high-quality medical care to middle and low income families in a clinic setting. The medical director, Dr. Connie Guion, continued as chief of the general medical clinic from 1932 to 1951. At that time, Dr. David Barr obtained a grant from the Commonwealth Fund of New York to establish the Comprehensive Care and Teaching Program in order to improve the teaching and practice of ambulatory patient care. Dr. George Reader, as director of this program, planned the reorganization of the outpatient department and the fourth-year curriculum to permit students to follow patients throughout the 22-week student clerkship in the general medical and pediatric clinics and obtain consultations without referring patients out. Students were encouraged to understand the social and psychological aspects of medical care, and through the Home Care Program they began to apply these principles in the community. The Comprehensive Care and Teaching Program also provided a meeting-ground for clinicians and social scientists interested in the social and administrative aspects of medicine and of medical education.[2]

The New York Hospital–Cornell Welfare Medical Care Project thus grew out of these fundamental interests of the city and the hospital. The Project further reflected the conviction that it is only through the synergy of public and voluntary agencies that services can be most effectively rendered to the people who need them. The traditional responsibility of the voluntary agency is to experiment with methods that can then be applied more widely by the public agency. As stated in the original grant proposal,[3] the experiment was performed so that it might "serve as a model for the establishment of Welfare family panels throughout the city."

Historical Background

Before the 1930's, the medically indigent patient was dependent upon the largely unsupervised and erratic charity of medical care institutions and private doctors. In small towns and rural areas facilities were sparse. In the large cities, there were clinics for the medically indigent, but those in teaching institutions were closely geared to educational rather than patient need, and those with no teaching

2. G. G. Reader and M. E. W. Goss, eds., *Comprehensive Medical Care and Teaching: A Report on the Establishment, Development, and Evaluation of the New York Hospital–Cornell Medical Center Program* (Ithaca: Cornell University Press, 1967).

3. "A Proposal for Demonstration and Study of a Complete Medical Care Program for Welfare Families," p. 1.

affiliation were often of low quality. Private doctors provided some free care, but the evidence suggests that this did not nearly meet the need.[4]

The inundation of the relief rolls during the depression revealed the fundamental inadequacy of private resources to meet the community's demand for medical care. The 1931 Wicks Act in New York State provided state reimbursement for the main elements of medical care for the indigent. The following year a nationwide system was established which permitted state and local payment (with partial federal reimbursement) for some of the elements of medical care for welfare recipients. It was left to the state and the local communities to decide which services should be provided, and these varied widely from state to state.

New York State (including New York City) provided a more complete range of services than most other states. But many different organizations were involved in giving care. They tended to operate independently, with minimal inter-agency communication and with individual administrative autonomy. New York City in the 1930's already had a large number of clinics providing free care, but they were enormously overcrowded and the care provided was usually poor. The Wicks Act, in planning medical services for the people on Home Relief (in 1934 there were about 600,000 out of a population of approximately 6,000,000, that is, 10 per cent of the population on Home Relief), stated that people should attend these clinics if they were able to travel; but for the first time clinic care would be supplemented by doctor home visits. The state Temporary Emergency Relief Administration would reimburse the city for sending doctors to the patient's home for "acute minor house-confining illnesses." There was no problem in finding doctors, because their income had been slashed by the depression; about 4,500 of them enrolled and were reimbursed $2.00 per house call.

There were many problems with the system, one of which was to prevent its abuse without regulating it so that it would be entangled in bureaucratic red tape. One of its most significant shortcomings, however, as pointed out by Dr. Mack Lipkin, then director of Welfare Medical Services for Manhattan, was the total lack of coordination between the patient's different sources of care. (We are indebted to Dr. Lipkin, who is now on the staff of the New York Hospital, for this discussion of welfare medical care in New York City during the depression.) If a child had an earache, for instance, he might first be taken to a clinic. If the earache persisted, the family might summon a welfare

4. For example, Harry H. Moore, *American Medicine and the People's Health* (New York: D. Appleton & Co., 1927); H. M. and A. R. Somers, *Doctors, Patients and Health Insurance: The Organization and Financing of Medical Care* (The Brookings Institute), 1961).

panel physician. If it developed into a mastoid, the child would have to be hospitalized, probably on the ward of a city hospital. In the course of this one illness, the child would have seen three doctors. The chances of their communicating with each other were negligible. Dr. Lipkin proposed a system of coordinated care, at the center of which would be, in each neighborhood, a well-qualified and well-paid doctor (working half-time) having a hospital affiliation and thus able to see the same patient in office, clinic, home, or hospital ward. This plan ran into opposition, however, and was never tried in practice.

Since the 1930's there has been a considerable increase in the number and range of facilities available to the indigent; but there has been little change, through the years, in the pattern of dispensing medical care. The system, like charity, its predecessor, has recently become anachronistic as its inadequacies have become more and more apparent. Its lack of coordination in administering services allows duplication and waste of time, energy, and money and makes it difficult to control or evaluate the effectiveness and quality of care.

Medical advances have added another dimension to the problem. The primary focus of American medicine has been on the study of acute illness. Highly specialized, basic-science-oriented laboratory medicine flourishes within the hospital, whose wards are used to provide a constant, acutely ill population for study. However, progress in the control of acute illness is now moving the attention of the teaching and research centers toward the study of common chronic diseases in the community. In the general hospitals, too, the primacy of acute illness has diminished and the ward census reveals an increasing proportion of aged and chronically ill patients. This gradual shift in focus is, however, only recent. Though the teaching and research center is still essentially insular in its commitments, the various community agencies, led by health and welfare departments, are forced to handle the additional social and economic problems created by the increase in chronic disease.

In 1958, definitive action was taken in New York City when the Departments of Health, Welfare, and Hospitals "began a joint undertaking to review and improve health services and medical care for recipients of public welfare."[5] This undertaking began with the creation of the position of deputy commissioner of welfare medical care, with an appointment on the staffs both of the Health and Welfare Departments and with direct access to both commissioners. Attention was focused on structurally reorganizing the existing program so as to try to improve the general level of welfare medical care. The medical

5. Baumgartner and Dumpson, "Health in Welfare," p. 1073.

center was viewed as a logical source of leadership; and the New York Hospital–Cornell Medical Center accepted the opportunity to pioneer in providing an organized program of welfare medical care.

A review of existing conditions revealed some of the multiplicity of sources from which New York City welfare clients could receive medical care. These included out-patient clinics of both city and voluntary hospitals, the emergency and in-patient services of these hospitals, the Home Medical Service of the Department of Welfare, proprietary nursing homes, and various other medical care resources. Many of these institutions were known to operate independently. In particular, it was known that neither hospitalization nor home medical care were necessarily coordinated with out-patient care.

As originally formulated, the problem seemed to be primarily one of patients fragmenting their own care, that is, attending several clinics simultaneously or switching from one to another during the course of an illness. This could mean that costly records, X-rays, and laboratory examinations at one clinic might be repeated needlessly at another. The phenomenon of the so-called "clinic shopper" was believed to be a frequent one. With the vision of hindsight, the trouble with the existing system of welfare medical care seemed to lie more with the organizational structure than with the patient. Its crucial weakness was that, with rare exceptions, no one doctor or group of clinicians undertook continuing responsibility for the indigent patients who came under their care. Whatever the reasons, the manifest lack of coordination of care, with its effect on quality of medical care, was a primary source of concern both to the Department of Welfare and to the New York Hospital. It was agreed that a system of coordinated medical care could be expected to be more effective.

The Project Proposal

Against this background, the New York Hospital–Cornell Medical Center, in cooperation with the Health and Welfare Departments of New York City, planned and established a demonstration project in welfare medical care. A contract was drawn up between the New York Hospital and the Department of Welfare for the care of a group of welfare recipients. A five-year grant was obtained from the Health Research Council of New York City starting July 1, 1960. Included in the grant funds were salaries of the clinical coordinating team, which was based at the New York Hospital. The aims of the Project, as formulated in the original grant proposal were: (1) to demonstrate that it is practical for a general hospital to provide complete medical care to welfare clients; (2) to study the utilization of services by welfare clients in the demonstration group and to compare this with the utilization of a control group who continue under the existing welfare medical care system;(3) to determine the costs of care under the two systems and to attempt to arrive at a reasonable capitation fee; and (4) to attempt to compare quality of care under the two systems.

Systems of Medical Care

A group of welfare clients in the Yorkville welfare district on the east side of Manhattan were offered medical care through the facilities of the New York Hospital, and a similarly selected control group was left to obtain care under the existing system. A special staff composed of physicians, nurses, and social workers provided and coordinated the care of those members of the study group who came to the New York Hospital. In addition to medical personnel, this special staff included a research team of sociologists, accountants, and others to study the experimental system and compare it with the existing system. The elements of service offered to the study group at the New York Hospital were the same, with minor exceptions noted below, as those available to welfare clients under the existing system, the difference being that they would all be offered under the auspices of one medical center rather than being available from many different sources.

Present Welfare Medical Care System (Control Group)

Up to a point, welfare medical care is synonymous with indigent medical care. Most indigent New Yorkers obtain their ambulant care in the out-patient clinics and in the emergency rooms of municipal and voluntary hospitals. When these patients require hospitalization, the Department of Hospitals pays in whole or in part for every person who can establish his inability to pay; one does not have to be on welfare to receive this financial assistance. Hospital-based home care services are also available at some hospitals.

For well-baby care, including examination and immunizations, but excluding treatment for illness (with the exception of one or two centers where experiments are being conducted in combining preventive and therapeutic services to babies and young children), Department of Health clinics are available without a means test. The Health Department also runs chest clinics (for tuberculosis) and venereal disease clinics, where patients are carefully followed and contacts investigated. Some district health centers operate diagnostic clinics, health maintenance clinics, coronary clubs, obesity clinics, and other special services. All these are preventive or diagnostic in nature; with a few exceptions, no treatment is given. (Exceptions include tuberculosis and venereal disease treatments and rehabilitation services for handicapped children.)

Dental care is provided by the School Health Service in school clinics and for children up to the age of twelve in Health Department dental clinics. Adults can have oral surgery (and sometimes prophylactic treatment) in dental clinics in hospital out-patient departments. For fillings, dentures, and so on, private clinics such as the Guggenheim provide some free care.

Mental illness is the responsibility of the state, once the patient needs long-term institutionalization, and the state-run system of aftercare clinics follows certain patients after discharge from the hospital. For short-term hospitalization, there are psychiatric wards in several voluntary and city hospitals. For out-patient psychiatric care, there are a number of clinics run under different auspices, but their capacity is quite limited.

The person newly admitted to welfare is encouraged to use these various facilities. But, in addition, he is entitled as a welfare recipient to some extra services not available to him when he goes off relief. The most important of these are as follows:

The Welfare Department pays a panel of doctors to make home calls on welfare recipients. In addition, a panel of specialists is available for domiciliary consultations, and laboratory services for patients ill at home are available on the request of a panel doctor. Welfare panel physicians are reimbursed only for home visits, not for office visits. A welfare client who wants a doctor calls his local welfare center and the clerk in the medical section assigns him a panel physician if he does not already have one. Thereafter, he may call the doctor directly.

The Welfare Department runs its own dental clinics, which give regular care including fillings, extractions, and dentures. Dental care, which is limited to oral surgery, is also available to those too ill to leave home.

In New York City, Welfare also runs its own eye clinics, which are authorized to refract the eyes and dispense glasses.

Welfare is naturally interested in assessing ability to work, or its converse, disability. When a client may be eligible for relief under the Aid to the Disabled category, medical evidence is needed in preparing the evaluation form, which the state will review. It is often difficult to obtain sufficiently accurate or prompt information from the hospital where the patient has been receiving care; the department has established special hospital-based clinics where such a preliminary examination, either for employability or for disability, can be performed.

The Welfare Department reimburses hospitals for out-patient care to welfare recipients, so that it is possible for voluntary hospitals to care for more welfare recipients than might otherwise have been the case.

Drugs prescribed in out-patient clinics are supposed to be furnished by the hospital as part of the services included in the visit, but drugs prescribed by the panel physician in the course of a home visit are paid for separately by the Welfare Department.

When the visiting nurse service is used for welfare recipients under the direction of a welfare panel physician or a hospital doctor, it is reimbursed by the Department of Welfare.

Welfare pays for the support of needy patients in nursing homes, and supervises their care through welfare panel physicians, who are obligated to visit them at specified intervals.

Bus or subway fare to take the patient to clinic is allowed for in the client's budget, and taxi fares may be paid for by welfare in certain circumstances. A telephone may be placed in the client's home on certification of medical need.

The Welfare Department pays for appliances such as dentures, eyeglasses, hearing aids, prostheses, and braces; equipment such as wheelchairs; and services such as homemakers.

Experimental Medical Care System (Study Group)

The following services were offered to the study group by the New York Hospital–Cornell Project: out-patient services; emergency services; home visits; home care; hospitalization; nursing home care.

Out-patient Service. It was planned that the patients would receive most of their care in the existing out-patient clinics of the hospital. A Project staff of physicians (internists and pediatricians) would give the care in the general medical and pediatric clinics and would coordinate the care given in the specialty clinics and elsewhere in the hospital. As an extension of present out-patient service, all Project patients would be eligible for care without question, bypassing the usual screening of new patients by the admitting residents. Well-baby care would be available in the general pediatric clinic; and certain extensions of service were made available in the areas of eye and dental care.

Emergency Service. In medical emergencies, and when the clinics were shut but the patient needed to be seen at the hospital, he could be brought to the emergency room at the New York Hospital. If an ambulance were needed, it was to be secured through regular police department channels. Project staff members were available to meet emergencies at the hospital or in the patient's home; at the hospital, they would work in conjunction with the regular emergency room staff.

Home Visiting. Project physicians would have the status of welfare panel physicians and would have authority from the Welfare Department to make home visits at the discretion of the Project, without prior authorization. Visiting nurse service was also available for home visiting in the usual way, under doctor's instructions.

Home Care. A home care service, extending hospital service into the home and offering 24-hour coverage, was already in existence at the New York Hospital. Project patients would be eligible for this service if they met the admission requirements. The most important of these were that they live reasonably close to the hospital and that the home be suitable for the needed care. If the patient needed regular home visiting but was not eligible for home care, the Project physician would make the home visits.

Hospitalization. The New York Hospital offered hospitalization to all patients meeting reasonable standards for admission to the hospital, for a period of up to two months. Patients needing long-term hospitalization would be cared for in other appropriate facilities, but would still be followed by Project physicians.

Nursing Home Care. Several nursing homes within the New York Hospital area were designated for the care of appropriate Project patients. The Project physicians would visit these patients and direct their medical care.

Thus, the services offered at the New York Hospital were designed to replace much of the existing system: out-patient and emergency visits at city and voluntary hospitals; acute hospitalizations not exceeding sixty days; home and nursing home visits from the welfare panel physicians; child health station visits; and much of the dental, eye, and psychiatric care.

Other services could not be offered directly, but Project staff hoped to refer patients to appropriate facilities, to keep in touch with the patients, and to resume contact when these services ended. Examples would be chronic hospitalization, admissions to mental hospitals, restorative dental services, and some psychiatric clinic care.

The precise extent to which the Project would be involved with other agencies on behalf of its patients was not known in advance, because the "existing system" only became known to Project staff in the course of the demonstration. One could learn on paper what services were theoretically available to welfare recipients. However, only experience showed which of these services were so rarely used as not to pose a problem of coordination and which were used so extensively that the Project had to try to evolve new ways of working with them in order to carry out its mandate of coordinating medical care. Some of these innovations in clinical liaison are described in Chapter 7.

Contract

Under the present system the Welfare Department pays for the medical care of its clients in various ways. For in-patient admissions to city or voluntary hospitals it reimburses the Department of Hospitals.

Voluntary and city hospitals are reimbursed (the latter through the Department of Hospitals) for clinic but not for emergency room visits. (When the Project began, the payment for a clinic visit was $5.00.) An elaborate system of prior authorizations and subsequent auditing controls medical expenditures in such areas as home visiting, drugs, appliances, and other items of medical cost.

To avoid the complexities of the existing administration of medical services, authority was delegated to the Project to initiate and control services such as home and nursing visits, visiting nurse service, drugs prescribed outside the hospital, eyeglasses, appliances, and patient transportation between hospital and home. Arrangements were made to pay for most of these on a capitation, rather than a fee-for-service, basis. During a pilot run the monthly capitation rate was based on actual Department of Welfare expenditures per case in the previous year. These ranged from $2.50 per case on Aid to the Blind to $3.00 per case for Aid to Dependent Children.[6] Once the Project had accumulated enough experience with the pilot group of patients, a new rate was negotiated, still using the Department of Welfare scale of reimbursement per service but based on utilization rates derived from the Project's own experience. The resulting capitation rate of $4.00 per case, regardless of welfare category, remained in effect for the duration of the Project.

6. For details see Appendix to the *Annual Report of the Project to the Health Research Council, 1961–1962.*

There is a long tradition of clinical investigation in medicine. Such research is usually carried out under the leadership of a "clinician" directing a research team. The modern model for this type of activity is found in the divisions of a department of medicine such as gastroenterology, hematology, or infectious disease. Each division concerns itself with its specific field of interest with appropriate basic scientists as well as clinicians participating. Within the teaching hospital it devotes itself to the tripartite goals of service, teaching, and research, and outside the hospital it relates to its scientific peer groups. It was with this kind of model in mind that the team of clinicians and social scientists assembled to carry out the work of the New York Hospital–Cornell Welfare Medical Care Project.

Modern clinical investigation cannot be carried out within the medical center without including appropriate basic scientists as part of the investigative team. In the examples cited above, it is normally the biological scientist with whom the clinician collaborates. Research into the delivery of health services to patients in the community, however, requires another kind of expert, the behavioral or social scientist. The medical care research team, therefore, includes clinicians and social scientists.

Sir William Osler once said that every discovery in the medical laboratory stemmed directly from a bedside observation by the clinician. This need for continuous interchange of experience between the clinician and basic scientist is particularly apparent in medical care research. The social sciences have only recently been extended into the field of health and medicine. Many of the initial studies during the last ten to fifteen years have been carried out by social scientists observing behavior within the medical center, but without close collaboration with physicians. Physicians sometimes fail to recognize the relevance of these early studies to the pragmatic problems of medical care. For this reason, a medical care research team with physicians and sociologists working in collaboration may be particularly fruitful now in building up the body of knowledge needed for the long-range solutions of medical care problems.

Development of the Clinical Organization

During the first year of the Project (July 1960 through June 1961), the primary task was to set up within the New York Hospital and the Department of Welfare the procedures needed to care for and study the group of patients selected and to evolve a research design that would include comparison of study and control group systems of medical care.

The medical care research team that was recruited to develop this program included internists, pediatricians, nurses, social workers, sociologists, statisticians, and accountants. During the year, the clinical staff worked toward integrating the care of the Project patients into the medical and pediatric clinics of the New York Hospital and setting up the methods of evaluating that care. At the same time, headquarters for the research team was established in the Kips Bay Health Center.

Particular emphasis was placed on establishing the Project within the regular structure of the New York Hospital. It was planned to base the care of the adults and children in the general medical and pediatric clinics, even though, at the time, these were separated from each other by three floors and several wings of the main hospital building. (In the following year, the general medical clinic was moved to new quarters on the same floor as the general pediatric clinic, but it was still a considerable distance from it.)

In the adult clinic, Project internists assumed the care of some welfare clients currently attending the clinic, so as to experience the kinds of problems that might be specific to welfare patients as distinct from other clinic patients. (Only about 9 per cent of the clinic patients in general medicine are welfare clients.) In the pediatric clinic, one of the pediatricians carried out a chart study on the medical records of children on welfare, randomly selecting 100 from among those currently attending the clinic. This study, which is described in Chapter 8, gave a picture of the medical problems of these children and formed a comparison group for the Project children later on.

Evolution of the Research Design

To fulfill the aims of the grant proposal, a number of measuring instruments had to be devised and administrative routines developed. The research was characterized from the beginning by the closeness of the clinical-social science collaboration. This extended to equal participation in designing the experiment, setting up the tools to measure it, and interpreting the results. It was the responsibility of the social scientists to randomize the experimental subjects into study and control groups, to devise valid measuring instruments, to control the quality of the interviewing, to build codes, process the data, and so on. At the same time, it was the task of the clinicians to devise the experimental system of care to be offered to the study group, to decide on the rate and method of intake of patients into that system and on the geographic area that could be served. In each phase of this developmental year there was a constant interchange of ideas and information, as the social scientists began to learn about the welfare process and the characteristics of the local indigent population and the clinicians developed medical care experience with the pilot group of welfare clients. These discoveries in turn led to continuous modifications in the study design.

The evolution of the plan of study may best be considered under the following headings: the nature of the sample, and the timing and method of intake of patients into the study; study of feasibility within the New York Hospital; the kind of instruments to be used in measuring utilization of medical services by study and control groups and in determining patient satisfaction; the method of measuring cost; the ways in which to compare effectiveness of medical care.

Broadly speaking, there were three stages of learning about the population to be studied before the design of the demonstration was finally crystallized. First, an analysis was made of all Department of Welfare statistics, including those from special studies the department had made from its own records. Second, a new study of welfare records was carried out. Third, there was a "dress rehearsal" of the entire process, in the form of a pilot run.

The Sample. From the beginning, the Project was a practical demonstration as well as an experiment, so the sample design could not be based on purely mathematical considerations. It was patently impossible for one hospital in New York City to offer to take care of a random sample of those of the city's inhabitants on welfare; some geographic limits would have to be set, thus making the Project into a local study rather than one rigorously representative of the city as a whole. Fortunately, citywide statistics on the welfare population were to make it easier to identify and to allow for local variations.

The New York Hospital's traditional district in the Yorkville area of Manhattan has become increasingly an area of luxury housing, as old tenements are torn down and replaced by high-rent apartment houses. There is practically no city-subsidized housing in the area. For this reason, the welfare district in which the New York Hospital is situated is a large one; it extended, at the time the Project started, from 6th Street in the south to 106th Street in the north, and from the East River to Fifth Avenue. Welfare clients would be likely to cluster at the extremes of the district, rather than near the New York Hospital.

A decision had to be made whether to try to cover the whole Yorkville district or only part of it and then whether, within the area selected, to take all the people currently on welfare or to invite new admissions as they came on the welfare rolls. Third, the rate and method of intake of patients into the Project had to be determined.

To help resolve these problems of sample size, area, and rate of intake and, in general, to learn as much as possible about the population the Project was to serve, the Welfare Department's routine statistics for New York City were reviewed. Some special investigations carried out by the department were also examined; but it soon became clear that a new study of welfare records would have to be made. In particular, there were three kinds of information needed that were not available from any existing source. First, it was necessary to find out where, within the local welfare district, most of the prospective patients lived. Second, in order to estimate the number of families the New York Hospital doctors could handle each month, it was important to have at least some idea of what medical care was reported under the old system. Third, to make a final decision on sample size, an estimate had to be made of how stable a population was going to be served. The Welfare Department's statistics, designed for fiscal and administrative purposes, were entirely cross-sectional and provided no longitudinal perspective of what happened to people and families over the course of time.

A cohort of cases newly admitted to welfare in the Yorkville district early in 1959 was selected and a total of 374 cases located and tabulated. (Preference in planning by this time was for new admissions rather than a cross-section of the welfare caseload, because it would permit a cleaner sampling design and would be less disruptive of ongoing medical care.) About half turned out to be readmissions, and half were on welfare for the first time. The chart study gave valuable information on the characteristics and the reported medical care of the cases. As had been suspected, they were indeed clustered at the northern and southern extremes, and very few clients lived near the New York Hospital. It was learned that of 1,000 welfare cases, just over half would probably be single-person cases on Old Age Assistance, Aid to the Disabled, or Home Relief. About half would be fairly large family cases, mainly on Aid to Dependent Children. In all, one could expect about 2,400 or 2,500 people in 1,000 welfare cases. About half of all the cases had medical care reported for them in the course of a year.

By far the most valuable aspect of the chart study, however, was the new form it gave to the original conception of the nature of the population group the Project was to serve. Instead of a welfare "population" that would atrophy somewhat over two or three years of care and study, the chart study disclosed a group of medically indigent people constantly crossing the line between total indigence and limited self-support. The prospect was that if 1,000 welfare cases were offered medical care to be paid for by welfare when they first came on assistance, less than half would still be on welfare two years later; and less than a quarter would have been on continuously. Some cases, especially those on Home Relief, would have received assistance for a very short time and then not again during the next two years. Even in Old Age Assistance, which one would expect to be a stable category, many cases would have closed during that period of time -- some of the closings being, of course, due to death. The pattern typical of Aid to Dependent Children presented the least stable picture and the one potentially most disturbing to continuity of medical care. These cases tended to close and reopen constantly, often at very brief intervals. Even when cases remained on welfare there were constant changes in status, such as transfers from one district to another, changes of welfare category, and alterations in case composition. The amount of clerical work involved at the Welfare Department in all these transactions was enormous.

Faced with this unstable situation, the Project had two alternatives; it could keep close to its original mandate of improving *welfare* medical care and ignore what happened to the patient when he went off welfare; or it could ignore the patient's welfare status and, once having offered him complete medical care, making it available to him indefinitely. There was little hesitation in choosing the second alternative. The prospect of caring for and studying a population in constant movement affected every aspect of the New York Hospital Project from then on. First, it suggested the necessity of securing adequate baseline data, because it might be hard to keep track of the population. Second, if the families included in the cohort study had been on the welfare rolls less than half of the two years which had been studied, then the medical care as reported in their records accounted for only part of the medical care actually received during the two year period. One could, therefore, not rely on welfare records as sources of utilization data. Moreover, the volume of medical need in the welfare population was very likely greater than generally estimated, and consequently a slow Project intake would be necessary so as not to overload the clinic facilities.

The financial problem was the next to arise, because of the turnover on the welfare rolls; and this also had repercussions on the research. Because payment for medical services was to be on a capitation basis, with the money coming from the Department of Welfare, questions arose about payment for clients off welfare altogether or in between welfare admissions. (Of course, one could never know at the time whether a particular case would reopen during the existence of the Project.) There was no legal barrier to the Welfare Department's paying the medical bills for medically indigent people off relief, but there was understandable reluctance to do so on a large scale. There was a legal precedent in the "medical services only," or "MS," category of payment; and the Welfare Department, in an effort to solve the financial problems that would result from the anticipated turnover, did invoke this "MS" category and write it into the procedures for the New York Hospital–Cornell Project. (However, the Welfare Department was unable to find a way to reimburse the hospital for the care it gave to patients during periods when they were not on public assistance.) The Welfare Department was less able to help with the problem of clients transferring from one district to another. Even if the patients had been willing to travel and the doctors to extend their home visiting territory, the administrative problems of following cases still on welfare but living in other districts would have to be left to the clinical and research staff of the Project; the Welfare Department's liaison procedures would not cover these cases.

Study of Feasibility at the New York Hospital. As foreseen in the grant proposal, the best demonstration of the practicability of providing complete care to welfare clients would be the successful establishment of the Project itself. This would need careful documentation. Preparations were therefore made during 1960–61 to identify Project patients and to record all the special services to be performed by the Project, such as home and nursing home visits, disability evaluations, disbursement of carfare, 24-hour telephone coverage, and so on. It was discovered that precise utilization of regular hospital services -- clinic visits, admissions, X-ray and laboratory visits, and so forth, could best be recorded by yearly review of the medical chart. Plans were made for medical audit of the charts, and members of each professional discipline -- internal medicine, pediatrics, psychiatry, social service, and nursing -- prepared to describe and summarize their experience with the patients they would see.

Originally, plans were made to keep track of each patient's welfare status on a day-to-day basis. The local welfare center would send a copy of the DRAT (Daily Record of Action Taken) to the Project each day, and an attempt would be made to keep Project records constantly up-to-date as to whether the patient was on or off welfare, had changed category, moved to another district, and so on. As will be seen later, this record-keeping was achieved during the intake period but eventually proved to be an insuperable task. A more realistic form of liaison with the Welfare Department was gradually evolved by the social service coordinator.

Meanwhile, the precise design of the clinical experiment was being worked out by the medical staff. One important need in studying feasibility was to know as much as possible about the health of the welfare population. This need led to a very important decision, which altered the original study design. Consideration had been given at one time to subjecting all members of the study group, not just those who could be persuaded to come to the New York Hospital, to some form of multiphasic screening examination, involving such procedures as chest X-ray, blood test, urinalysis, and so on. This did not really seem to be possible, however; nor was it felt that this was the best way to learn about the general health of patients who did not come to the New York

Hospital voluntarily. The physicians believed that good medical care involved taking a complete history and physical examination, no matter how localized the patient's complaint and that, although a small number of laboratory procedures and X-rays might be useful routinely, most of these should be used judiciously and at the discretion of the doctor.

It was therefore decided to try to give a complete medical examination rather than a multiphasic screening to a randomly selected sample of welfare clients. It was known that this would be more expensive in the short run because it would involve persuading people who would not otherwise have seen a doctor to do so at least once. However, in order to permit a fair comparison with the control group, some of the study group would have to be left to seek medical care in their own way, when they saw fit. The study group was therefore divided in half; half would be left to come for medical care when they thought it was needed, as under the existing system, and for the other half, an appointment for a complete examination would accompany the invitation to the New York Hospital. Those receiving an appointment were designated the "appointment," or A group; the others the "demand" or B group.

Measuring Use of Services and Patient Satisfaction in the Two Systems. In order to investigate total use of medical services, and attitudes to the care received, it was clear that both study and control group members would have to be interviewed at intervals during the experimental period. Because there was the critical problem of keeping track of the clients, it became not merely desirable but essential to have baseline interviews. The first wave of interviews was therefore planned to take place immediately before Project intake, that is, for study group members just before their invitation to the New York Hospital and for control group members just before they became eligible for welfare medical care under the existing system. The second and third wave interviews would be administered as nearly as possible one year and two years after the baseline interview for each case.

Three areas needed to be covered in the original questionnaires if these were to provide as much assistance as possible in understanding what later happened in the medical care experiment. First, a health questionnaire would give comparable information on members of the study and control groups about health status at intake. (Though the health of the study group members who came to the New York Hospital could later be studied much more thoroughly and accurately than by questionnaire, this would not be true of those who did not come nor of the control group.) This health questionnaire, for members of the study group, would also serve as a systematic review for the Project doctors and save time when the patient came to the New York

Hospital. It was also desirable to know something about the medical care the clients had used in the past, both as a way of describing the patients (as high or low utilizers, as accustomed to clinic or private doctors, and so on) and as a way of getting leads on where they might go in the future if they needed a doctor. A utilization questionnaire was therefore written, asking which hospitals in New York City respondents and their families had ever attended and concentrating particular attention on the medical care received in the last 12 months.

Both the health and the utilization questionnaires asked factual questions, so it was felt that the setting in which they were administered was not too likely to interfere with the answers. These questionnaires were therefore administered by the Project staff in the Welfare Center. For questions on attitudes, however, it was felt that the home was the more appropriate place for the interviews and that it would be important to have them conducted by an organization that was clearly not connected with either the Welfare Department or the New York Hospital. The National Opinion Research Center (NORC), affiliated with the University of Chicago, but with offices in New York, was retained for this purpose.

The attitude questionnaire explored four main areas before the Project began: the feelings of the patient about medical care in general, his attitude to doctors and other health personnel, his proneness to seek medical care, and his image of the various hospitals in the neighborhood. It seemed desirable to know what the welfare recipient valued most in medical care: skill, friendliness, convenience, continuity, accessibility, or some other attribute and to know whether he had different priorities for different situations (emergency or otherwise, for instance) or for different members of the family. It would be of interest to know what he thought about doctors in general; what kinds of doctors he personally preferred; what he thought doctors could do for him, if anything; and whether or not he thought clinic doctors and private doctors behaved differently. It would also be useful to know his experience with nurses and social workers and his feelings about them and other hospital staff. It was necessary to know which people were eager to go to the doctor (and perhaps happy to try a new hospital) and which ones customarily put it off as long as possible. Opinions about the stage of an illness at which one needs care and the best place to go for different conditions - private doctor, clinic, emergency room, or some other place – might also affect the response to the Project. Lastly, information was wanted on whether or not the people about to be invited to the New York Hospital had heard of it or attended it before and, if so, what opinion they had of it.

These questions seemed to cover the topics that would most directly affect the respondent's behavior in the Project. There were many others that could profitably have been asked, and some were tried out in the pre-test; but practical considerations, including costs, suggested that a one to one and a half hour interview would be sufficient.

Measurement of Cost. From the outset of the experiment, it was evident that costs could only be measured precisely within the New York Hospital. The services of Arthur Andersen & Co. (the regular auditors of the New York Hospital) were obtained for the purpose of developing standard costs for the various services utilized by Project patients within the hospital.

Because the Project patients were offered all the elements of care normally provided for the hospital's "ward" or "clinic" population, a complete cost study of the hospital, starting with the original engineering drawings and allocation of space, was considered necessary. The base period used in the development of the standard cost data was January 1, 1960, to June 30, 1960. Adjustments were made for this six month period where abnormal circumstances were noted, for example, where amounts reflected in the accounting records were not representative of approximately one half of the annual totals shown in the hospital financial statements. (The information and the methods used in developing standard costs for the various services offered by the hospital are discussed in detail in Chapter 9.) To complete the cost comparison of the two systems of care, it was necessary to develop the best figures available from public records and reports of the other institutions involved in the study and control group care. Because the accuracy of these data does not approach that of the New York Hospital data, however, comparisons must be made guardedly.

Comparing Effectiveness of Care under the Two Systems. The aim of measuring quality or effectiveness of care was cautiously stated in the original proposal for several reasons. First, this task is in general notoriously difficult. Second, in a welfare population medical care may be only a small part of the service needed to show any improvement in function. Third, two years may be too short a time to show results. Nevertheless, plans were made for investigating the deaths in study and control groups, for comparing pre-natal and post-natal experience, and for examining the reasons for and duration of hospitalization in the two groups. In addition, the health questionnaire was viewed as a starting point for quality of care comparisons. Respondents in study and control groups reporting a particular symptom or set of conditions at intake could be followed through their medical records, both within the Project and outside it, to see if they had received care for this condition and what kind of care they had received.

Pilot Run

In order to test all the procedures and research tools and to uncover potential diffficulties in the provision of medical care, a pilot run was carried out in the spring of 1961. Preparations were not really complete, but no further delay was possible if the demonstration was to start on time on July 1 of that year and if one were to take advantage of all the lessons to be learned in the pilot run.

For five weeks Project interviewers were stationed in the Yorkville Welfare Center, and as people were accepted for public assistance, letters were sent to them to return to the center for an interview. When the clients returned, an interviewer administered the health and utilization questionnaires. If by random selection the person or family belonged to the control group, the interview was then complete. If he fell into the study group, the Project was explained to him after the questionnaires were administered, and he was invited henceforth to obtain all his needed medical care at the New York Hospital. A brochure explained how to get to the hospital, how to reach a doctor at night, and so on. Half the study group members (the B group) were given the brochure only and were left to seek care as they felt the need. The other half of the study group (the A group) were given the brochure and also a clinic appointment, one for the adult to the general medical clinic and one for the youngest child to the pediatric clinic. (If there was more than one adult, the appointment went to the "case-head," that is, the person to whom the welfare check was made out. Other family members were to be brought in after these first visits.)

The response to the invitation was encouraging. Even though many lived some distance from the New York Hospital, most of the 176 pilot cases invited did come. By the beginning of July, three to four months after the invitation, at least one case member was seen by a Project physician in 81 per cent of the cases given appointments, and 45 per cent of the demand group had also made contact with the hospital. Careful records were kept of the response patterns, and in the fall an analysis was made of the total experience with this group of patients. In fact, members of the pilot study remained a pilot group throughout the life of the Project, and each successive wave of questionnaires was pre-tested on them. (The people in the pilot control group, C group, were used only for pre-testing questionnaires. No medical follow-up of this group of 96 welfare cases was done.)

Revision of Procedures

During May and June of 1961, procedures were revised on the basis of the pilot run experience. The health and utilization questionnaires would have to be given when the client first applied for welfare, rather than after acceptance, because the latter procedure had caused serious delays in making medical care available to the new recipients. The home interview would have to be fitted as smoothly as possible into an already complicated set of intake procedures to minimize such delay. Once the home interview was completed and the Welfare Department had authorized the patient's care at the New York Hospital, the head of a study group case would receive a letter of invitation to the Project on a Department of Welfare letterhead, together with the New York Hospital brochure.

In the meantime, a manual of procedures was assembled. This included a definition of the study population; explanation of the relevant welfare terminology and procedures; the proposed method of intake into the Project and details of the procedures to be followed after intake – such as how to provide ambulance service, reimburse for carfare, work with the visiting nurse service, and so on. Finally, a complete set of letters, questionnaires, and forms evolved by the Project staff was appended. This manual of procedures proved to be an important tool for communication and coordination of activities among staff members and with outside agencies.

Intake to the Project

By dint of great effort, all was in readiness to begin the Project on July 1, 1961, as scheduled. Interviewers from the Project moved into the Yorkville Welfare Center and began administering the health and utilization questionnaires in English and Spanish to all applicants for public assistance. Practically none of the applicants refused to be interviewed, although in very rare instances the completion of the interview was impossible for practical reasons. A completion rate of 99.0 per cent was achieved on the health and utilization questionnaires, so that the baseline data in this area are virtually complete.

When the first person applying for relief in the Yorkville district after July 1 was accepted on welfare, his case was referred to the National Opinion Research Center for the home interview. At first, the procedure of getting the eligible study group case onto the Project was somewhat protracted; the first family did not officially enter the demonstration until July 20. But as the difficulties were ironed out, this interval was greatly reduced, and eventually the lag between acceptance on welfare and invitation to the Project for the study group averaged only five days.

When the patient appeared at the hospital and was identified as a Project patient, he was allowed to bypass the normal hospital screening procedure and come directly to the Project desk in the medical and pediatric clinics. In the medical clinic, the patient was assigned to one Project internist who would henceforth be his doctor; in the pediatric clinic, the three pediatricians took care of the patients interchangeably.

The NORC interviewers had numerous adventures in securing the home interviews. Respondents lived in some of the worst areas of the city, many in rundown tenements, transient hotels, or flophouses. Although the interviewers had a street number for the respondent, there was often no indication of where in the building he lived; mailboxes were without names, doors sometimes unnumbered, corridors ill-lit. Neighbors tended to be suspicious and not inclined to cooperate in tracing the designated respondent. Mainly because of the skill and tenacity of the interviewers, a completion rate of 98.1 per cent was achieved on the home interviews, which exceeded the most optimistic hopes.

The problem was not that respondents were reluctant to be interviewed at home but was usually one of locating persons; hostility was encountered in a very small number of instances. In fact, in the judgment of the interviewers, less than 3 per cent were actually "hostile or suspicious."

The paperwork involved in processing cases into the Project was fully as great as had been expected, especially for cases in the study group, whose medical care at the New York Hospital had to be authorized by the Welfare Department. The predictions about the extent of duplication of cases in the total "cases added" in the Yorkville district in the course of a year and about the proportion of ineligibles to be expected, were fulfilled within very narrow limits. (Ineligible were out-of-district clients, residents of old age homes, and those who did not remain on welfare long enough to complete intake to the Project.) Aiming at a study group of 1,000 welfare cases and a control group two thirds that size, intake ended with a yield of 1,681 cases instead of 1,667. Random allocation into A, B, and C groups resulted in 538 A group cases, 491 B group cases, and 652 C group cases. Intake ended on June 30, 1962, although another six weeks elapsed before the last eligible applicants were processed into the Project.

First Year on the Project

Because intake into the Project was staggered over a twelve-month period, all later interviews were similarly staggered. Even before the last person had been interviewed on the first wave of questionnaires, it was time to approach the first people entering the demonstration in order to find out what medical care they had received during the last twelve months and to solicit their opinions of this care.

The first question to be settled was precisely which people constituted the sample for this second interview. The original sample consisted of those persons who were members of each welfare case at the time the case was accepted on the project, with one adult (chosen at random if there was more than one in the case) speaking for the case as home interview respondent. But in the course of a year, as the chart study showed, many changes would have taken place in the case constellations. Aside from the obvious changes occasioned by births and deaths, there would be instances in which an original welfare case was split into two or more new ones, or in which two original cases were amalgamated. Many cases would, of course, be closed, so that one could not say what would have happened to the case constellation had its members remained on welfare.

This flux in the basic analytic unit, the welfare case, presented challenging problems in sampling. It was finally decided to "freeze" the population for research purposes as it was at intake and to investigate the medical care received by all those persons who were case members at that time. No one would be dropped from the study and the only persons added for research purposes would be babies born to members of the original welfare case. (To avoid hardship to families and fulfill obligations to the Welfare Department, persons added to an original study group case were eligible for medical care on the Project, but they were not included in the research.) For the attitude questionnaire, the same home interview respondent would be kept throughout, allowing no substitutions.

Only one interview per case was planned for the second wave. Questions were constructed to record the use of medical services by the respondent and the other members of his welfare case. The respondent was then invited to express his opinion about the care they had received and to state in general how this year's medical care compared with that received during the previous year. As many as possible of the questions on general attitudes to doctors, hospitals, and so on, that had been used in the first home interview were repeated in order to allow tracing over time any changes in those attitudes that might accompany experience with one or another system of medical care.

One new series of questions which was included in the second wave questionnaires and which proved extremely effective was a set of direct questions about coordination of care. Coordination is a key theme of this research, and one of its main purposes has been to find out why people go to more than one hospital and why there is often so much apparent duplication in services received. It had been thought that this could be studied only by observing behavior and not by asking questions about the matter. But, because of the articulateness and common sense that was found to an unexpected degree in the answers to the first home interviews, it was decided to ask the patients direct questions. Where respondents reported using more than one hospital or seeing both a private doctor and a clinic doctor, they were asked why this had occurred. Furthermore, they were asked which hospital or hospitals they intended to use in the future; and if they listed more than one, they were asked why this was so and under what circumstances they would use each one.

The problem of finding the people to be interviewed was much more difficult in the second wave. The chief reason for this, of course, was that nearly half of the respondents were no longer on welfare, and so for them no up-to-date address was available from the Department of Welfare. The second wave completion rate of 80 per cent (85 per cent if those who had died, moved away, or become institutionalized are excluded) of the whole population reflects, on the one hand, the tenacity of the interviewers and the comparative ease of finding those clients still on welfare, and on the other hand, the above-average mobility of the group no longer on welfare but still indigent.

Second Year on the Project

The third and final home interview, like its predecessor, was taken into the field in the month of August as the previous wave was being completed. For questions on the use of medical services the original population was again the one covered (as well as babies born to members of the original welfare case); for questions about health and for the attitude questions the same home interview respondent was again approached.

For each respondent, this interview would end the two year experimental period under one or the other of the two systems of medical care; it was thus possible to ask members of the study group if they had received an invitation to the New York Hospital Project and if they had gone there. Those who acknowledged going were asked what they liked and disliked about the Project; those who said they did not go were asked why not. All respondents were asked if they considered one place as the main place to obtain their medical care and if they had one doctor they considered their own doctor. All were asked where they intended to go in the future if they needed medical care.

Documenting Utilization of Services

At the New York Hospital, the medical records of those patients who responded were abstracted in detail to show the month-by-month use of services. Moreover, in order to pick up those patients who had indeed come to the hospital but through some mishap had never reached the Project staff, the name of every member of the study group was checked more than once through the hospital record room files. Data on response to the invitation are thus believed to be virtually complete.

Utilization of medical services outside the New York Hospital was far harder to document. The last two waves of home interviews were designed primarily to provide information on the source of care used. The patient was asked to report the number of times he had visited a clinic, been admitted to a hospital, and so forth; but these estimates were to be checked, as far as possible, against the actual records of the hospital used. Details on how this was done are provided in Appendix D.

3 | The Project Population:
Social Characteristics and Welfare Status

New York City Welfare Population

When intake to the New York Hospital Cornell Project began in July 1961, there were 345,772 people on welfare in New York City, grouped into 140,421 cases (see Table 1). They were on welfare for four main reasons. The largest group was families with dependent children under 18, in which there was no breadwinner. There was a single parent -- nearly always the mother -- who was widowed, divorced, separated, deserted, or unmarried, or her husband was sick or disabled or institutionalized. The category of Aid to Dependent Children, created by the Social Security Act of 1935, supports such cases. (Originally only the children were supported. In 1950, provision was made in the budget to include one parent.) In mid-1961, nearly two thirds of the people and more than a third of the cases on relief in New York City were on Aid to Dependent Children.

The next largest group of people were the elderly, aged 65 or over, receiving Old Age Assistance or Medical Aid to the Aged. This former category of public assistance also dates back to the Social Security Act of 1935. Medical Aid to the Aged, which gives assistance to the medically indigent for medical bills but does not provide basic support, is of very recent date. Implementing the Kerr-Mills Act of 1961 it first went into effect in New York City in April 1961, only three months before Project intake began.

1. Public assistance caseload in New York City, July 1961.

Category	Welfare cases Number	Welfare cases Per cent	Persons Number	Persons Per cent
Aid to Dependent Children	50,545	36	209,587	60
Old Age Assistance Medical Aid to the Aged	32,860 } 10,347 }	31	32,860 } 10,347 }	12
Aid to the Disabled Aid to the Blind	24,163 } 2,149 }	19	24,163 } 2,149 }	8
Home Relief	15,897	11	40,257	12
Temporary Aid to Dependent Children	4,460	3	26,409	8
Total	140,421	100	345,772	100

The third group of people eligible for assistance were the "totally and permanently disabled" on Aid to the Disabled, a category created in 1950. Certification of disability by a State Review Team is necessary to qualify for this category; welfare clients awaiting such review are classified as "Pending Aid to the Disabled" (PAD). In July 1961 they, together with the small number of blind persons supported by a separate relief category, contributed about one fifth of the New York City caseload but were less than 10 per cent of the persons on relief.

These three groups of welfare recipients -- the dependent children, the old, and the disabled -- are supported by federal categories of relief. Assistance is administered through the states, and the federal government reimburses part of the cost through matching funds.

The fourth group of people on public assistance -- the unemployed -- are largely on Home Relief. For these cases there is no federal reimbursement. Home Relief cases may be either individuals or families. The single recipients often suffer from limited education or intelligence or from lack of work skills; some have disturbed personalities or disabilities that may one day qualify as "total and permanent" but have not as yet done so. Families on Home Relief may be receiving supplemental assistance only, in instances where the wage earner is working but not earning enough to support his family.

In July 1961, federal reimbursement was extended to some families with children where the wage earner was unemployed or not earning enough; the federal category of Temporary Aid to Dependent Children was created, and eligible cases were transferred to it from Home Relief. Toward the end of the Project experimental period, in November 1963, this federal support became permanent, and the former Aid to Dependent Children and Temporary Aid to Dependent Children were combined into Aid to Families with Dependent Children. However, the terms ADC and TADC are still employed.

In contrast to the welfare caseload, the cases newly admitted to welfare in July 1961 show a reversal of the relative positions of Home Relief and Old Age Assistance (see Appendix Table A-1). Although Old Age Assistance constituted almost a third of the caseload, it was only about one tenth of the new admissions, so it seems to be a relatively stable category that builds up slowly and has relatively little turnover. Home Relief, by contrast, represents a very large number of short admissions to welfare.

The New York Hospital–Cornell Project Population

With a change of focus from the city as a whole to the Project population, Table 2 shows the number of persons and cases, drawn from new admissions to welfare in the Yorkville district, who entered

2. New York Hospital Project population: cases and persons by study group.

Group	Welfare cases		Persons	
	Number	Per cent	Number	Per cent
A (appointment)	538	32	1,331	32
B (demand)	491	29	1,173	28
C (control)	652	39	1,685	40
Total	1,681	100	4,189	100

the New York Hospital–Cornell Project and fell by random selection into the A, B, and C groups. The original intention was to achieve a 30:30:40 distribution, so the A group is slightly over-represented vis-à-vis the B group. The major variables have been checked for comparability in the A, B, and C groups, and a summary of this information will be found in Appendix Table A-2. Henceforth in this chapter, background characteristics will be presented for all study groups combined, with the understanding that there are only random variations between them.

The people in the Project population can be described and grouped in many different ways. In fact, one of the perennial problems has been the determination of the unit of analysis. To the Welfare Department they were *welfare cases* and, because this was the original sampling unit, it was one that could never be ignored or superseded. To the hospital they were sick *individuals*, traditionally divided into children under 14 seen in the pediatric department and adults 14 or over seen in the medical department. The study was carried out with the collaboration of the Health Department, interested in the health of the community and accustomed to dealing with families or *households.*

The interrelationship of these three units – welfare case, individual, and household -- is exceedingly complex. It has posed many problems for the clinicians giving care because the system of frequently dividing families into two or more welfare cases has greatly complicated the delivery of family care; and it has created endless problems for the research staff in data processing.

To begin with the welfare case and individual, Table 3 shows the kinds of groupings that made up the 1,681 study and control group welfare cases. Half the cases consisted of a single adult. Nearly all the rest contained children under 18, with the pattern of a single parent and children predominating.

The welfare category of the single cases is shown in Table 4. They are almost evenly divided into the aged, the disabled, and the single unemployed. Many of these single Home Relief cases either have a past

3. Project population by case constellation at intake.

Constellation	Welfare cases		Persons	
	Number	Per cent	Number	Per cent
Single adult	848	50	848	20
Mother and children[a]	483	29	1,632	39
Husband, wife, and children	275	16	1,521	36
Father and children	31	2	102	2
Related adults[b]	29	2	63	2
Children only[c]	15	1	23	1
Total	1,681	100	4,189	100

[a]Always with some under 18.

[b]Eighteen were husband and wife, 8 were mother and adult child(ren), 2 were husband and wife with adult children, and 1 group contained a brother and sister.

[c]Eleven were single-child cases.

4. Welfare category at intake of the single-person cases.

Category	Number of cases	Per cent of all cases
Old Age Assistance	288	17
Medical Aid to the Aged		
Pending Aid to the Disabled		
Aid to the Disabled	305	18
Aid to the Blind		
Home Relief — single cases	255	15
Total	848	50

history of disability investigation (having been on Pending Aid to the Disabled but rejected for that category of relief by the State Review Team), or else, if the experience of similar cases is borne out, they will end in the Aid to the Disabled category. (In the study of welfare records described in Chapter 2, Home Relief cases were often found to end on Aid to the Disabled.) It is for that reason that they are grouped with the other single-adult cases, rather than with the Home Relief family cases, for most of the analysis.

In Table 5 family cases are described by welfare category at intake. This table shows that although only half the *welfare cases* on the project were multi-person cases, four fifths (80 per cent) of the *individual persons* belonged to such cases. Appendix Table A-3 combines Tables 4 and 5 and shows the distribution by welfare category of all the cases and persons on the Project.

The average number of persons per case was 2.5; and, if the single cases were excluded, the average per family case was 4.0. Thus, one was dealing with rather large families, and particularly with large families of children. Those with the most children tended to be constellations of husband, wife, and children, although there was quite a sizable minority of very large families in which the mother was the only adult in the case. There were rarely more than two and never more than four adults in the same case.

Welfare cases containing more than one person have been described interchangeably as "multi-person cases" and "family cases." The latter term is not strictly correct, however, because the welfare case and the household unfortunately do not always coincide. First, the Project

5. Welfare category at intake of the multi-person cases.

	Welfare cases		Persons	
Category	Number of cases	Per cent of all cases	Number of persons	Per cent of all persons
Aid to Dependent Children	592	35	2,157	52
Temporary Aid to Dependent Children	146	9	747	18
Home Relief	95	6	437	10
Total	833	50	3,341	80

population did not necessarily include all those members of the household at intake, nor even all those on welfare in each household because, in order to preserve the "cleanness" of the sample, only cases that met the criteria of being newly accepted on welfare in the district during the intake year were invited to attend the New York Hospital. Second, many Project cases were known to be "mutual" to each other, that is, separate welfare cases living in the same household. Thus a single-person case like a man on Aid to the Disabled might not really be single but might be living with his wife and children; he might also be on welfare and on the Project, with the wife and children receiving a separate welfare check under the Aid to Dependent Children program. Nearly all these strands of red tape that entangle the average family needing public assistance can be traced to the rigidity and complexity of the eligibility requirements set by Congress for the various federal categories of assistance.

Ethnic Group. Table 6 shows the broad ethnic groupings of these people on welfare. The information was obtained from the home interview respondent, and it may not hold for all the other members, especially in families with children where several fathers are involved. The assumption has been made that where the respondent is Negro or Puerto Rican the other case members are also. (The term "Puerto Rican" is used here to mean "born in Puerto Rico" when adults are described and "born either in Puerto Rico or in the United States of Puerto Rican born parents" where children are concerned.)

The largest single ethnic group consists of Puerto Ricans who, although American citizens, are mostly comparatively recent arrivals in New York City. They have inherited the problems experienced by wave after wave of newcomers to the United States -- the language barrier, unfamiliarity with the city, lack of education, and lack of skills. Puerto Ricans predominate especially in the families on Temporary Aid to Dependent Children and Home Relief (Appendix Table A-4), where the main reason for needing public assistance is the inability of the parents to earn enough to support the family. Most of the persons on Aid to

6. Project population by ethnic group (total persons).

Group	Number	Per cent
Puerto Rican	2,319	55
Negro	739	18
Non-Puerto-Rican white	1,131	27
Total	4,189	100

Dependent Children (where there is no employable breadwinner) are also Puerto Rican, although throughout the city many are Negro. (There happen to be few Negroes in the Yorkville district.) The single cases tend to contain white people of American or European origin; this is especially true of the oldest welfare clients, on Old Age Assistance and Medical Aid to the Aged.

Area of Residence. The Yorkville welfare district extended in July 1961 from 6th Street to 106th Street and from Fifth Avenue to the East River. (The boundaries actually changed during the intake year, and part of the northern area was added to the East End district. To preserve the integrity of the sample, the Project interviewers invited East End cases in the area formerly belonging to Yorkville to the Yorkville Center for interview and even sent an interviewer into the East End Center one day a week for the last few months of the Project intake.) New admissions to welfare, as Table 7 shows, were very unevenly distributed within the area. To make simple categories of home address, the Yorkville district was divided into east-to-west slices, combining streets so as to yield the most homogeneous groupings in terms of ethnic group of the respondents, proportion of single and family cases, and (for the study group) response to the Project invitation. Nearly three quarters (72 per cent) of the individuals were clustered at the two extremes of the district, either on the Lower East Side below 14th Street or in East Harlem above 96th Street. This tendency was particularly observable in the family case members, very few of whom lived near the New York Hospital. Only 12 per cent of the total population lived in the New York Hospital district between 57th Street and 95th Street; and district patients formed 25 per cent of the single-person cases but only 9 per cent of the family case members.

7. **Project population by address at intake, distinguishing single- and family-case members (total persons).**

Address	Single-case members		Family-case members		Total persons	
	Number	Per cent	Number	Per cent	Number	Per cent
6th–13th Street	197	23	1,247	37	1,444	34
14th–29th Street	187	22	310	9	497	12
30th–56th Street	73	9	86	3	159	4
57th–95th Street	214	25	286	9	500	12
96th–106th Street	177	21	1,412	42	1,589	38
Total cases	848	100	3,341	100	4,189	100

Convenient sources of medical care for the people at the northern end of the Yorkville welfare district would be Metropolitan Hospital at 98th Street and First Avenue and Mount Sinai at 100th Street and Fifth Avenue. Those on the Lower East Side would be closest to Bellevue Hospital, on First Avenue between 25th and 29th Streets.

Neighborhoods in large cities tend to display sharp ethnic differences; the Yorkville welfare district in Manhattan is no exception to this rule. Table 8 shows the relationship of address at intake to the broad ethnic groupings of the persons in the Project population. Its shows that Puerto Ricans newly on welfare divided rather evenly between the

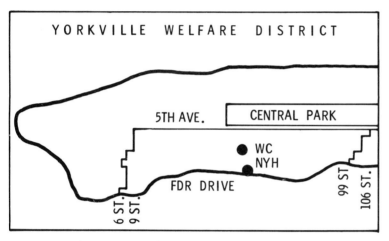

Fig. 1. Map of Yorkville Welfare Center district

8. Project population by address at intake and ethnic group (total persons).

Address	Puerto Rican		Negro		Non-Puerto Rican white		Total	
	Number	Per cent	Number	Per cent	Number	Per cent	Number	Per cent
6th–13th St.	1,031	44	145	20	268	24	1,444	34
14th–29th St.	251	11	30	4	216	19	497	12
30th–56th St.	29	1	12	2	118	10	159	4
57th–95th St.	84	4	17	2	399	35	500	12
96th–106th St.	924	40	535	72	130	12	1,589	38
Total	2,319	100	739	100	1,131	100	4,189	100

northern and southern clusters (with slightly more in the south of the district); the Negroes were concentrated above 96th Street; and the non-Puerto Rican white recipients predominated in the central area, especially around the New York Hospital.

The interrelationship of the three factors -- address at intake, ethnicity, and membership in single or family welfare cases -- is shown in combination in Appendix Table A-5. The importance of these factors will become apparent in later chapters when the response of the study group to the invitation is discussed.

Education. As might be expected, these people on the whole did not have much education (see Table 9). Nationwide, 28 per cent of the population over 18 graduated from high school and went no further, and another 18 per cent have gone beyond high school to college.[1] The corresponding figures for the Project are 10 per cent of home interview respondents who were high school graduates without college and another 7 per cent with some college education. Eight per cent of the adults interviewed had no schooling at all, compared with only 2 per cent of adults in the nation.

The question "Do you feel that you had a chance to get as much schooling as you wanted?" was used in the interview as a tactful way of

9. Education of home interview respondents.

Grades completed	Number	Per cent
None	100	8
1–3	145	11
4–5	159	12
6–7	177	14
8	203	15
9–11	303	23
12	132	10
More than 12	91	7
Total	1,310[a]	100

[a]This question was asked on the second home interview, after welfare records had failed to supply complete data on education. Of the 1,681 respondents, 1,310 were interviewed on the second wave and answered this question.

1. *Statistical Abstract of the United States, 1964.* U.S. Department of Commerce, Bureau of the Census, Table 147, figures for the year 1962.

obtaining the information on the exact number of grades completed; but it also provided a sidelight on the respondents themselves. There is naturally a correlation between the answers to this question and the amount of schooling they had—those who had the least were the least satisfied with the amount they had received—but there was a large number of people with very little formal education who expressed no desire to have had more.

There are significant ethnic differences in education, too. The median number of years of schooling was 9 and a half for Negroes, 5 and a half for Puerto Ricans, and 7 and a half for non-Puerto-Rican whites. The fact that the Negro on welfare has the most schooling of the three groups suggests the strength of the barriers other than education or skills that operate against him in the struggle for economic advancement. The Puerto Rican, the most recent immigrant, has been to school the least.

Religion. The great majority of the people on the Project were Catholic. Altogether, 66 per cent of the home interview respondents said they were Catholic, 24 per cent said they were Protestant, 3 per cent belonged to the Hebrew religion, 3 per cent to other religions, and 4 per cent to none.

The three baseline questionnaires administered before intake -- the health, utilization, and attitude questionnaires (see Appendix B) -- were designed to help answer three questions: What was the health of these people at intake? How were they accustomed to obtaining their medical care? How did they feel about health, illness, doctors, and hospitals? The health questionnaire was administered to the 1,980 adults who were aged 18 or over at intake. The attitude questionnaire was addressed to the one adult from each welfare case who had been designated as the home interview respondent (1,681 respondents). The bases in the tables in this chapter will therefore vary according to whether the question is a "health" question (base 1,980) or an "attitude" question (base 1,681 or the 1,643 of them who were successfully interviewed).

Health Status

Adults, it will be remembered, were interviewed with the health questionnaire in the welfare center, usually on the day they first applied for assistance. In a quarter of the cases it was not possible to intercept them at the center (or they could not come in person because of age or illness), and the interview was done at home by NORC personnel after administration of the attitude questionnaire. In 80 per cent of all health questionnaires, the person answered for himself, in 14 per cent his spouse answered for him, and in the remainder some other relative did so. Each person was asked if he now had, or had had in the past, any of 30 specific illnesses and then if he had recently observed or presently had any of 31 symptoms. Finally, he was asked if any health conditions interfered with his life in four areas of functioning.

Illnesses. Appendix Table A-6 shows the replies to the questions about illnesses. The outstanding feature of this table is the first entry: no less than 47 per cent of all the adults on the Project considered that they "suffered from nerves" and, for practically all who answered positively, this was a present rather than a past illness at the time of intake. Sinus trouble, reported less than half as frequently, was the next most common present or past condition, with high blood pressure a close third; but if past illnesses are left out, then both of these are outranked by arthritis and varicose veins.

Reported illnesses naturally vary greatly by age: Appendix Table A-7 shows present illnesses by broad age groupings. It is apparent that "suffering from nerves" is a complaint that ranges over all age groups, with no particular age-specific pattern except perhaps a peak in the forties. Even teenagers (18 to 20 year olds) complain of it in over a third of the cases. Arthritis, heart trouble, and varicose veins show the expected correlation with age.

In order to test the reliability of the health questionnaire in a general way, the Project physicians reviewed the original health questionnaires on about half the adults who came to the New York Hospital; for each illness they signified if they thought the patient had it at intake, had had it in the past but not then, or had never had the illness. Altogether there are 255 questionnaires in which both doctor and patient have responded to questions about present and past illnesses. These 255 questionnaires each contain responses to questions about the 30 illnesses (adding up to a total of 7,650 responses). Table 10 shows that, for this particular set of conditions, if the patient says he has a condition, the odds are almost 2 to 1 that he does so far as the doctor can determine; if he says he does not have a condition, the odds are close to 24 to 1 that he is right. To use the doctor-patient agreement legitimately, however, one must look separately at the different conditions; naturally, the agreement varies widely from one to another. Appendix Table A-8 shows that agreement was good in those "suffering from nerves." In 130 instances, patient and doctor agreed that the patient "suffered from nerves." In another 10 cases, this was the patient's opinion only, but in a further 27 instances the doctor thought this condition existed, although it had not been mentioned by the patient. In other words, the evidence suggests that there is indeed an extremely large group of patients who "suffer from nerves";[1] far from

10. Reliability of patient responses to the health questionnaire in a sample of patients seen by Project doctors (255 patients).

Responses	Number	Per cent
Illnesses checked "yes" by patient		
Doctor agreed	556	62
Doctor disagreed	341	38
Total	897	100
Illnesses checked "no" by patient		
Doctor agreed	6,521	96
Doctor disagreed	237	4
Total	6,758	100

1. The Midtown study found 58 per cent of all those interviewed in a probability sample of New Yorkers to be characterized by mild to moderate symptom formation, with an additional 23 per cent described as "impaired." Srole, Leo, et al., *Mental Health in the Metropolis: The Midtown Manhattan Study*, I (New York: McGraw Hill Book Co., Inc., 1962), p. 138.

exaggerating the number, the health questionnaire may in fact under-report those who could be so classified.

There was very little disagreement between doctor and patient regarding thyroid disease and prostate trouble. The patients tended to over-report sinus trouble, rheumatic fever, and ulcers but to underreport arteriosclerosis and cancer. The number of cases of anemia changes little from patient's report to doctor's version, but there is little agreement on who it is who is anemic. The same is true of diseases of the kidney or bladder. Agreement was best, aside from the category of "suffering from nerves," in cases of asthma, lung trouble, tumor, female disorders, and varicose veins.

Symptoms. Appendix Table A-9 shows how symptoms were reported by the 1,980 adults in the study and control groups. Again, the apparent amount of psychiatric and emotional difficulties is impressive; symptoms that suggest this were more frequently reported than any others except localized problems, for example, tooth decay and eye trouble. Nearly half of those reporting were "very depressed and blue recently," and almost as many (often the same people) were "tired all the time." Headaches, backaches, insomnia, and poor appetite were very common, and many patients were continually troubled with aches and pains. Potentially serious organic problems are not excluded either: there are plenty of symptoms suggestive of heart disease, tuberculosis, cancer, and other major illnesses. The impression is one of many sick, unhappy people.[2]

When the symptoms are viewed by age group (Appendix Table A-10), a consistent phenomenon becomes apparent. Whatever the patterns of symptomatology by age group -- whether a steady rise with the years or a series of ups and downs -- there is almost always a decline in symptoms reported past age 65. This was even apparent in many of the illnesses shown in Table A-6, but it is more pronounced with the symptoms. Most other surveys have shown increasing morbidity and disability with advancing age, greatest of all in the 65-and-over age group.[3] Here again, the selective mechanism of the welfare process

2. Factor analysis was performed on similar self-report items in a questionnaire of the National Mental Health Survey. A factor that includes nervousness, trouble with sleeping, headaches, and loss of appetite was iterated and labeled "a conscious distress state" or "psychological anxiety." Gerald Gurin, Joseph Veroff, and Sheila Feld, *Americans View Their Mental Health* (New York: Basic Books, 1960), p. 184. The fact that most of the health questionnaires were administered at the welfare center at the time the respondent applied for public assistance lends validity to responses that depict a conscious distress state.

3. For example, Ray E. Trussell and Jack Elinson, *Chronic Illness in a Rural Area: The Hunterdon Study*, III, *Chronic Illness in the United States* (Cambridge, Mass.: Harvard University Press, 1959), pp. 156-164.

seems the likeliest explanation for this discrepancy. People over 65 go on welfare because they are old; they do not necessarily have to be sick also to qualify. But in the forties, fifties, and early sixties an increasing proportion of welfare recipients are actually or potentially disabled -- that is mainly why they are on welfare -- so that there is an unusual amount of illness among people in these age groups. (It will be remembered that the younger age groups are made up mostly of women needing support because they have dependent children.)

One other factor that might help account for the drop in symptomatology in the oldest clients is that the Project was unable to accept those entering old age homes because medical care was already provided there and could not be paid for twice. New admissions to Old Age Assistance on the Project were thus drawn from among those still living in their own homes and were therefore likely to be healthier than other members of their particular generation.

Self-evaluation of Health. When asked to rate their own health and that of their spouse and children as excellent, good, fair, or poor, home interview respondents tended to be less optimistic than the average person. This particular question has been used several times in past NORC surveys, so that comparisons with other populations are possible. An survey[4] in 1955 of a national sample of adults found far more positive estimates of health than were found in the Project patients, and so did a 1959 study[5] of eighteen to sixty-five year old adults in selected non-rural areas. The 1955 comparison is particularly pertinent because it covers all age groups, whereas the 1959 study excluded old people and therefore might be expected to report better health. The comparisons are shown in Table 11.

Table 12 shows the comparison for respondents' evaluation of their spouses' and children's health. (These questions were not asked in the 1959 study.) The same kind of difference between Project patients and a cross-section of the country is again apparent. It is particularly striking that practically all parents in the general population rate their children's health as excellent or good (92 per cent) but only 64 per cent of the Project parents do so. There are differences within the Project population, however (Table 13). It is principally the members of the single welfare cases who rate their health as poor. (This difference can be explained in part by the fact that ill health is frequently the criterion

4. Survey 367, National Opinion Research Center. The study, entitled "The National Study of Attitudes toward Health and Medical Care," was done for the Health Information Foundation, an organization now affiliated with the University of Chicago. Jacob J. Feldman *"The Dissemination of Health Information"* (Aldine Publishing Company, Chicago: 1966) draws on much of the data from this study.

5. U.S. Department of Health, Education, and Welfare, "Attitudes toward Cooperation in a Health Examination Survey," *Health Statistics,* (Washington, D.C., July 1961), series D-NO, 6.

11. Project respondents' self-evaluation of health compared with two national samples (in per cent).

Health rating	Project respondents (N=1,643)	1955 study (N=2,362)	1959 study (N=762)
Excellent	9	30	31
Good	29	38	45
Fair	38	25	20
Poor	24	7	4
Total	100	100	100

12. Project respondents' rating of health of spouse and children compared with national sample (in per cent).

	Spouse		Children	
Health rating	Project patients (N=273)	1955 study (N=1,865)	Project patients (N=751)	1955 study (N=1,234)
Excellent	11	26	18	48
Good	38	41	46	44
Fair	32	25	31	7
Poor	19	8	5	1
Total	100	100	100	100

13. Respondents' rating of own health comparing single-case and family-case respondents.

	Single-case		Family-case		Total	
Health Rating	Number	Per cent	Number	Per cent	Number	Per cent
Excellent	65	8	81	10	146	9
Good	175	21	299	36	474	29
Fair	286	35	341	42	627	38
Poor	292	35	92	11	384	23
Don't know	6	1	6	1	12	1
Total	824	100	819	100	1,643	100

for assignment to the single person case, for example, Aid to the Disabled and Medical Aid to the Aged.) Respondents in family cases are not particularly enthusiastic about their own health, but tend to rate it in the intermediate categories of "good" or "fair."

Health Concern. Two questions in the first home interview explored the extent to which health occupied people's minds. Respondents were first asked if they thought about their own health fairly often, once in a while, or hardly ever and then how much they talked about their health. It is not surprising, in view of the illness reported above, to find that health is on their minds a good deal. Four groups of approximately equal size were distinguishable: the 23 per cent who both think about and talk about their health fairly often; the 28 per cent of "isolated worriers," who think about it fairly often but rarely discuss it; the 25 per cent with an intermediate level of concern; and 26 per cent who rarely give it a thought. When compared with national samples, the Project patients tend to show an understandably greater preoccupation with their health than the average person.

Disability. Certain cautions must be borne in mind in interpreting replies to the questions: "Do you have any illnesses or health conditions that interfere with your usual work? Your daily activities in the home? Traveling around the city? Going to visit family or friends?" The question did not work very well. It was intended to be the obverse of the physicians' rating of functional disability; but there was some misunderstanding on wording, and the patients raised such points as the fact that they had no social life anyway, so it was hard to say if it had been curtailed by illness. Table 14 presents the replies to the question about disability in the four areas listed above.

14. Disability reported by adults in four areas of functioning (in per cent, N=1,980).

Disability	Work	Other daily activity	Local travel	Social life
Great deal	24	7	15	12
Some	7	4	8	5
Little	5	3	5	3
None	64	86	72	80
Total	100	100	100	100

Past Medical Care

The next question to be asked involved the manner in which these patients had previously been accustomed to obtaining medical care. Had their many health problems been neglected, or had the patients been making many visits to the doctor? Were they used to the *kind* of care to be offered by the Project -- mainly clinic care, with home visits available but somewhat discouraged – or were they accustomed to seeing a private doctor in his office or having a welfare doctor come to the home for most of their care? Last, were they familiar with the experimental hospital?

The answers to some of these questions come out of the baseline questionnaires. But in a sense "the existing system" the Project tried to replace can be adequately described only in a full analysis of what happened to the control group. This detailed analysis is presented in Chapter 10. The impression gained from these initial interviews was that the volume of medical care used in the past was enormous. The rate of hospitalization appeared to be several times the national average, especially in the single-person cases. Many people had long hospital admissions. The great majority of general hospitalizations took place in the two city hospitals, Bellevue and Metropolitan, with more in the former than the latter. A small number of hospitalizations took place in each of a number of voluntary hospitals, with Mount Sinai and the New York Hospital in the lead among voluntary hospitals; but these accounted for only a small proportion of the total in-patient care.

Ambulant care, also apparently higher than the national average, was mainly concentrated in out-patient clinics and emergency rooms. Here again the two local city hospitals greatly predominated in the amount of care given. The New York Hospital had provided clinic care to a small number of patients (about 15 per cent had ever been there, half of these in the 12 months preceding Project intake); very few patients had used it for emergency care.

Thus the Project would be inviting for care a segment of the local population that was largely unfamiliar with the experimental hospital. Clear and explicit directions were needed on how to reach the New York Hospital and for simplifying intake procedures so that Project patients would not get "lost" once they did reach the admission unit. These considerations modified the evolution of procedures for Project intake.

The initial interviews disclosed that for every three patients reporting one source of care in a year there were two reporting more than one (though rarely more than two sources). Describing numbers of sources of care, however, is not the same as measuring coordination or its converse, fragmentation (see Chapter 10). It has become increasingly apparent, moreover, that one year is a very short time in which to assess coordination of care.

Attitudes to Doctors and Hospitals

The first home interview also explored some of the feelings, opinions, and attitudes of the population toward health and medical care. Attention was focused on those attitudes that might subsequently affect patients' behavior if they were invited to try a new system of care. Wherever possible, questions used in previous studies were included, so that comparisons could be made between this welfare population and either a cross-section of the American people or some other sub-group. It was expected that some of the attitudes toward medical care would change as a result of exposure to the Project. It was therefore necessary, as part of the experimental design, not only to obtain a general picture of the population at intake but to initiate a series of panel questions. By repeating these questions at the end of the first and second year of medical care, it would thus be possible to measure changes in attitudes that occurred under the two systems of care and to see what impact the Project had on those members of the study group who responded to the invitation (see Chapter 13).

Several attitudes toward health and medical care were investigated in the first home interview: attitudes relating to the organization of medical care; feelings about doctors and other health personnel; proneness to seek medical care; opinions about particular hospitals, especially the New York Hospital.

Organization of Medical Care. The interviewers sought to discover, among other things, the patient's general orientation to medical care facilities, including his future intentions about the kinds of facilities he might consider using, as well as those he had actually used in the recent past. One question listed a battery of conditions usually needing medical attention and asked what the respondent would do for each condition -- call a doctor, go to a clinic, or go to an emergency room. From the results it appeared that the patients were more inclined toward treatment in a clinic or emergency room than by a private doctor. In about half of all the instances, they reported that they would seek care for a given condition in a clinic (Table 15), and among the rest of the replies "go to the emergency room" slightly outnumbered "call a doctor." Respondents did not fail to differentiate between conditions, however: the emergency room, for instance, was chosen for treatment of unexplained weight loss of several months' duration by a low of 4 per cent of patients, and a high of 78 per cent said they would go there for a broken arm.

Patients could be broadly classified as doctor users, clinic users, or emergency room users. In the 100 cases, 51 respondents favored clinics, and 28 preferred private doctors. (The 100 cases are a randomly selected subsample of the first 500 welfare cases accepted into the

15. Facility respondents would use for certain conditions (in per cent, (N=1,643).

Condition	Call a doctor	Go to clinic	Emergency room	Don't know or other
Frequent stomach upsets	19	51	21	9
Varicose veins	16	68	7	9
A broken arm	9	11	78	2
Possible heart trouble	26	58	12	4
Nervousness	27	52	7	14
Troublesome boils	18	65	11	6
Feel sick all over	28	45	18	9
Spitting blood	19	32	46	3
Itching skin	18	67	9	6
Fever of 105°	21	11	63	5
Sleeplessness through worry	24	39	5	32
Unexplained weight loss	22	62	4	12
All conditions	21	47	24	8

Project's study group. They represent a 20 per cent subsample of the first 500 cases or almost 10 per cent of the entire study sample.) Only 10 mentioned the emergency room more often than they mentioned any other facility, but many mentioned it in conjunction with clinic use.

Within the 100 cases, those preferring private doctors seemed to be older, sicker, single-person cases of white American or European stock. Those apt to prefer clinics seemed to be family cases, usually Negro or Puerto Rican. A question on emergency medical care asked: "If you suddenly needed a doctor at night or on Sunday, what would you do?" The purpose of the question was to investigate the use of private doctors or welfare doctors (if the person had been on welfare before) compared with the use of institutional sources of help. The tendency was greatly in the direction of the institution: 44 per cent of respondents would go to an emergency room for medical care at night or on a Sunday, and 26 per cent would call the police or an ambulance (which would take them to an emergency room). Only 16 per cent would phone a doctor (and an additional 5 per cent would send someone to fetch a doctor).

Thus it turned out that clinics and emergency rooms were the main medical facilities these patients had used in the recent past; and they were the facilities to which most of them expected to turn for a wide range of conditions in the future. Moreover, it seemed that in many instances they actually preferred these institutions to private care. When asked "If you could choose, and it didn't cost you anything, would you rather go to a *hospital* clinic or emergency room, or would you rather see a private doctor?" 41 per cent of the respondents said they would rather go to clinic or emergency room. Thus in almost half the cases it did not seem to be only economic necessity that precluded private care.

Some of the reasons for preference are shown in Table 16. Some could have been predicted. Private doctors are preferred for interpersonal reasons (for example, "He takes more time with you. You can see he's more interested in you and wants to help you"), because less waiting is involved, and because it is more convenient. Clinics or emergency rooms are preferred because of the facilities they provide, or because they cost less, or because (unlike the private doctors, in the opinion of these respondents) they are not interested in your money. More competent medical care, though the votes may go to either side, is a frequent reason for preferring one or the other and is second only to interpersonal reasons.

A rather surprising response was the preference relating to continuity of care. Nine per cent of the respondents prefer a private doctor because they can always see the same doctor, but no less than 25 per cent of those preferring a clinic do so because they can see several different doctors. This is not merely a matter of having specialists

16. Distribution of preference for clinic or private doctor by reason given.

Reason	Prefer doctor (N=840)		Prefer clinic (N=671)		Total giving preference (N=1,511[a])	
	Number	Per cent	Number	Per cent	Number	Per cent
Interpersonal reasons	368	44	110	16	478	32
More competent medical care	184	22	204	30	388	26
Less waiting	345	41	23	3	368	24
Better facilities	26	3	233	35	259	17
One doctor (private)	74	9				
Many doctors (clinic)			167	25		
Cost considerations	30	4	117	17	147	10
Familiarity: I know them (him)	42	5	68	10	110	7
Familiarity: They know me	50	6	39	6	89	6
Availability	20	2	31	5	51	3

[a]The remaining 132 of the 1,643 respondents did not state a preference for clinic or private doctor.

available for consultation while one doctor provides continuity of general care; to judge from the comments, patients seem to feel several doctors are safer than one and that this consideration outweighs any desire for continuity.

The next question asked specifically: "When you go to a clinic, how important is it that you see the same doctor each time?" Table 17 shows the replies, separating those preferring private doctors from those preferring clinics. Those who prefer the former are more likely to value continuity than those who prefer clinics; but only a little over half of all the respondents endorsed continuity as "very important."

Attitudes to Doctors. A number of surveys have shown that most people are satisfied with their own medical care;[6] even those who are inclined to criticize doctors in general tend to approve of their own doctor and even to be very enthusiastic about him.

A question early in the questionnaire established that 77 per cent of the respondents had seen a doctor about their health in the last twelve months and that 76 per cent of these were entirely satisfied with the care and treatment they got from doctors during this period. However, when they were allowed the opportunities later in the interview to voice complaints in various areas, they were not unwilling to offer criticism. The respondents were presented with a battery of negative items about doctors and were asked whether or not they thought these items were true of most doctors; half agreed that: "They don't tell you enough about your condition; they don't explain just what the trouble is." More than a third (37 per cent) agreed that: "Doctors give better care to their private patients than to their clinic patients." Precisely one third agreed to the following propositions: "They don't give you a chance to tell them exactly what your trouble is," "They don't take enough personal interest in you," "They tell you there's nothing wrong with you when you know there is," and "Doctors rush too much when they examine you."

Another question listed possible attributes of doctors and asked the respondent to pick out the three or four that described the kind of doctor he himself liked best. Respondents picked old rather than young doctors in a ratio of more than four to one and men rather than women doctors by more than two to one. The choices are illustrated in Table 18. Again, the leading item had to do with adequacy of information about illness. Just as the leading criticism of doctors was that "They don't tell you enough about your condition," so the leading preferred attribute was that the doctor should "tell me all I want to know about my illness."

6. For example, "Social Surveys in Britain in 1956," quoted in Almont Lindsey *Socialized Medicine in England and Wales,* (Chapel Hill: University of North Carolina Press, 1962), pp. 230-231; Survey 367, NORC; Jacob J. Feldman *"The Dissemination of Health Information"* (Chicago: Aldine Publishing Company, 1966) p. 86.

17. Extent of respondents' desire for continuity, by clinic/doctor preference.

Importance of continuity	Prefer doctor		Prefer clinic		Don't know		Total	
	Number	Per cent	Number	Per cent	Number	Per cent	Number	Per cent
Very important	515	61	336	50	53	40	904	55
Fairly important	79	10	63	10	4	3	146	9
Not important	203	24	256	38	46	35	505	31
Don't know or no answer	43	5	16	2	29	22	88	5
Total	840	100	671	100	132	100	1,643	100

18. Distribution of doctor preference of respondents (N=1,643).

Attribute	Number	Per cent
Tells me all I want to know about my illness	980	60
Takes a personal interest	863	53
Extra thorough and complete	744	45
Speaks my own language	605	37
Puts me at ease	444	27
Spends a lot of time with me	281	17
Doesn't ask unnecessary questions	261	16
Tries not to give me too much medicine	155	9
Is my own religion	97	6

The largest number of respondents (38 per cent), when asked what they would most want the doctor to do for them in a hypothetical case of disabling backache, were concerned with finding out exactly what illness they had, and 16 per cent with whether or not it was serious. Nineteen per cent wanted the doctor to get them back to usual activities as soon as possible. Only a relatively small group (12 per cent) wanted immediate relief more than anything, and an even smaller group (8 per cent) seemed to accept it as inevitable and wanted to learn how to live with the condition.

In the literature[7] there is ample evidence of the communication difficulties involved when class barriers are crossed in the attempt by middle-class physicians to give medical care to lower-class patients. All the evidence available from the Project suggests that patients have a very real desire for communication with the physician.

Seeking Medical Care. Patients may perceive their symptoms or signs of illness and interpret them as such, yet fail to seek medical care. There is considerable variation among patients with similar conditions in their tendency to go to the doctor. In view of the high utilization rates of welfare clients, it was pertinent to seek any clues available on whether or not much of this was "unnecessary care," sought by people over-ready to go to the doctor for trivial reasons. The first attitude questionnaire investigated readiness to seek medical care by asking several questions in this area.

The most direct question asked was "In general when you're not feeling well, do you usually see a doctor right away; or do you wait for

7. For example, Kenneth R. Hammond and Fred Kern, Jr., *Teaching Comprehensive Medical Care: A Psychological Study of a Change in Medical Education* (Cambridge, Mass.: Harvard University Press, 1959), p. 40.

awhile, to see if it will go away; or do you usually put off seeing a doctor as long as you possibly can?" The answers to this question are shown in Table 19. The largest single group of respondents (44 per cent) took the middle-of-the-road position; but if they went to extremes, it was in the direction of putting off seeing a doctor as long as possible (34 per cent).

It was also of interest to know what kinds of conditions respondents thought needed medical attention. To help answer this question, a series of conditions was listed, ranging in seriousness from one as minor as "sore throat and running nose for a couple of days" to some of the seven classic cancer symptoms such as coughing up blood or an unusual lump on the body. Respondents were asked for each one if they would see a doctor right away, take care of it themselves, or leave it alone.

People are usually readier to say in an interview that they will see a doctor than they are actually to see one,[8] and the welfare clients seemed to be no exception. There was no condition for which less than 40 per cent said they would see a doctor right away, and for many conditions more than 80 per cent said they would (Table 20). But respondents were discriminating in their evaluation of which conditions needed attention most. Their ordering of priorities, from coughing up blood or lump on the body as most needing professional care, down to sore throat or constipation as least needing it, coincided almost exactly with the Project physicians' consensus about conditions they considered most in need of medical attention.

Some of the items in this question were used in the 1955 and 1959 surveys mentioned earlier, although sometimes the wording was a little different, which makes exact comparisons impossible. In general, Project respondents seemed *less* apt to see a doctor right away than people in the other samples; this attitude would tend to contradict the idea that they were seeing a doctor unnecessarily on a great number of occasions.

19. General readiness of respondents to see a doctor when not feeling well.

Response	Number	Per cent
See doctor right away	326	20
Wait a while	725	44
Put off as long as possible	559	34
Don't know	33	2
Total	1,643	100

8. Survey 367, NORC.

20. Distribution of responses about readiness to see a doctor for specific conditions (in per cent, N=1,643).[a]

Condition	See a doctor	Care for himself	Leave alone	Don't know
Coughing up blood	94	2	1	3
Unusual lump on body	93	2	1	4
Shortness of breath	83	7	4	6
Pain in chest	81	12	3	4
Bad cough for several weeks	77	18	1	3
Tired all the time, no reason	67	18	10	4
Frequent headaches	63	29	4	4
Feeling very depressed and blue	45	24	24	7
Sore throat, running nose, for couple of days	41	50	5	4
Diarrhea or constipation for couple of days	40	50	5	4

[a]Seven of the items used by Koos to explore respondents' recognition of symptoms that require medical attention are similar to items included in the Project's questionnaire. For each of the comparable items, at least 50 per cent fewer of Koos' Class III respondents (lowest socio-economic group) report the need for medical attention; for example, for the item "shortness of breath" only 21 per cent of Koos' group would seek medical attention, only 31 per cent would see a doctor for pain in the chest. (E. L. Koos, *The Health of Regionville,* New York, 1954, p. 32.) However, Feldman has pointed out the difference in wording in Koos' survey, in which only those who felt they would *invariably* see a doctor for the condition in question are entered under that column. Our findings are more consistent with other surveys cited by Feldman. (Jacob J. Feldman, *The Dissemination of Health Information,* Chicago: Aldine Publishing Company, 1966, pp. 60-64.)

In a cross-tabulation of Tables 19 and 20, there is a correlation between general delay pattern and stated reactions to individual conditions: respondents who seem in general to see a doctor readily say they would see a doctor right away for each condition with greater frequency than those patients who either wait a while or put off seeing the doctor (Appendix Table A-11). For those conditions that are manifestly serious, almost everyone, regardless of general delay pattern, would see a doctor right away. Differences between the three groups emerge only when comparison of readiness to see the doctor is made for such conditions as sore throat, depressed feeling, tiredness, bad cough, and frequent headaches.

If patients were apt to delay seeing a doctor when they themselves considered it necessary, it was desirable to discover some of the reasons for it. Was it lack of money? (In the immediate past no one had been on welfare, but they must have been very poor.) Was it practical considerations, such as a young mother's babysitting problems or a disabled person's difficulty getting on or off a bus? Or was fear of doctors or of hospitalization apt to discourage people from seeking professional help when they knew they needed it? The answers to these questions would be helpful in interpreting not only the original response to the invitation but later behavior – whether or not patients continued to come when they needed care.

Forty-one per cent of the respondents said they never did put off seeing a doctor when they thought they should; as for the delayers, Table 21 shows the reasons most often endorsed by them. (The responses were a series of reasons suggested by the interviewer, not a

21. **Distribution of reasons why respondents put off seeing a doctor (in per cent, N=1,643).**

Reason	Project patients	1955 study	1959 study
It's hard to go when I have children to look after	42[a]	–	–
I don't like to bother the doctor unless it's necessary	35	41	5[b]
I didn't want to spend the money on a doctor unless I had to	26	38	43
The doctor might want to put me in a hospital	19	–	5
I was too busy to see a doctor; I didn't have time	19	35	–
I didn't know any really good doctor	18	11	–
Traveling in the city is such a problem	14	–	–
I didn't think the doctor could help me any	13	9	5

[a]Per cent of those with children.

[b]Worded "unless I'm sick" instead of "unless it's necessary."

tabulation of free answers, so the reasons are said to be "endorsed" rather than "given.") These particular reasons were chosen from a number used in the 1955 and 1959 studies; and the wording used was exactly the same as that used in at least one of the surveys, so that comparison *can* be made here. Particular items were included in or excluded from the questionnaire on the basis of frequency of endorsement in the pretest.

The two items not previously used (referring to travel problems, in general and with children) were designed with a view to the fact that welfare clients lived some distance from the hospital and might find it hard to travel so far for the reasons suggested. These items were in fact often endorsed. In the others, the most striking difference between the Project population and those questioned in the national surveys was fear of hospitalization. This was mentioned by only 5 per cent of respondents nationwide and was last in order of frequency out of 18 possible reasons, whereas on the Project it was the fourth most frequent reason given for delaying and was endorsed by 19 per cent of the responents.

Some of the reasons given may be evasions -- particularly those suggesting the respondent was too busy or that he did not know a good doctor. Respondents endorsing these items might be classified as general "delayers" -- those who avoid seeing the doctor as a general rule and whose evasions may cover deep-seated reasons, which they do not voice, such as fear of illness or death, anxiety about separation from the family, and so on.

All these three questions on readiness to see a doctor -- what clients did "in general," what a person *should* do for particular symptoms, and reasons for delay that might have affected their past behavior -- were related to *general* tendencies and attitudes. The next question was a more specific one: "Suppose you were offered a free physical examination next week -- would you certainly go, probably go, or probably not go?" This question was asked because members of the appointment group *were* about to be offered "a free physical examination next week," and clues about what might deter patients from accepting the offer could be helpful in planning ways to improve the response to the invitation.

The attitude to adult physical check-ups was found to vary according to ethnic group. Table 22 shows the response of Puerto Ricans, non-Puerto-Rican whites, and Negroes, to such a (then) hypothetical offer. The great majority of the whole group expressed a willingness to accept the offer, but Negroes and Puerto Ricans were seemingly more willing to go than whites, a quarter of whom said they probably would *not* go.

If respondents were, by and large, enthusiastic about having a free physical examination for themselves, they were almost unanimous in

22. Distribution of responses to offer of a free physical examination, by ethnic group.

Response	Puerto Rican		Non-Puerto Rican white		Negroes		Total	
	Number	Per cent	Number	Per cent	Number	Per cent	Number	Per cent
Certainly go	567	80	443	63	176	75	1,186	72
Probably go	85	12	72	10	35	15	192	12
Probably not go	54	7	165	24	24	10	243	15
Don't know or no answer	4	1	18	3	0	—	22	1
Total	710	100	698	100	235	100	1,643	100

wanting this for their children: no less than 89 per cent would "certainly take them" if the offer were made to examine the children without charge. The actual response to the offer, as will be seen in later chapters, followed a very different pattern.

Opinions about Hospitals. The last set of attitudes systematically investigated before patients entered the Project related to opinions about local hospitals, with the image of the experimental hospital being of crucial importance.

The utilization questionnaire revealed that relatively few Project patients had ever been to the New York Hospital before and that even fewer had been there in the previous year. Eighteen per cent of the respondents mentioned it spontaneously in the course of the home interview in reply to the various questions about hospitals. Those who did not mention it of their own accord were asked directly, at the very end of the interview, whether or not they had ever heard of the New York Hospital: they divided exactly even on this question.

There were sharp ethnic differences between those who were and were not familiar with the New York Hospital. Very few Puerto Ricans were familiar with it. The Negroes had heard of New York Hospital two to one but did not mention it spontaneously when being asked about hospitals in general. To a great extent, it is a hospital known to the non-Puerto-Rican white population, a fact that reflects the general ethnic composition of the neighborhood surrounding the New York Hospital and of the patients attending its clinics.

When asked what they had heard about it, the great majority of the respondents gave replies that were favorable. They ranged from rather general, vague approval to extreme enthusiasm. Respondents were asked to which hospital(s) they would most and least like to go if they were completely free to choose. The ten leading hospitals chosen as either "most liked" or "least liked" are shown in Table 23. The New York Hospital ranks fourth in frequency of mention and ties for second place with Mount Sinai in the proportion of total mentions (93 per cent) that were favorable. Both these factors – frequency of mention and proportion favorable -- have to be borne in mind when assessing the image of a particular hospital.

These people had been accustomed to getting their medical care from the two big local city hospitals, Bellevue and Metropolitan. Bellevue evoked many criticisms but also inspired great enthusiasm and devotion. Metropolitan had patients devoted to it also, but it tended to attract more unfavorable remarks. Two other city hospitals -- Harlem and Lincoln -- were mentioned in an almost consistently negative light. A great number of voluntary hospitals were mentioned, nearly always favorably, with Mount Sinai and the New York Hospital heading this list.

23. Distribution of respondents' choice of hospital[a] (N=1,643).

Hospital	Total times mentioned	Would most like to use[b]	Would least like to use[c]	Liked as per cent of total mentions
Bellevue (city)	648	441	207	68
Metropolitan (city)	368	190	178	48
Mount Sinai	245	227	18	93
New York Hospital	160	149	11	93
Harlem (city)	96	3	93	3
Lenox Hill	88	79	9	90
St. Vincent's	79	72	7	91
Columbus	63	45	18	71
Columbia-Presbyterian	56	54	2	96
Lincoln (city)	52	2	50	4

[a]Showing the ten most frequently mentioned hospitals.

[b]Eighty-one respondents (5 per cent) did not name any hospital they liked most.

[c]874 respondents (53 per cent) did not name any hospital they liked least.

The respondents turned out to be more medically sophisticated than had been expected. Not only did they seem to know what symptoms should receive a doctor's attention, but they also tended to know rather clearly the advantages and drawbacks of the facilities available to them.

Two | **Experience within the New York Hospital**

5 | Response of the Study Group to the Invitation to the New York Hospital

The first concern in establishing the feasibility of providing complete care to a panel of welfare families was whether a sufficient number of them could be persuaded to attend the medical facility to which they were invited; the second concern was whether they would stay with it and use it as their main source of care.

The welfare record studies had shown that welfare clients in the Yorkville district were clustered mainly at the northern end, between 96th and 106th Streets, or at the southern end, between 6th and 14th Streets. The former were accustomed to obtaining medical care from Metropolitan and Mount Sinai Hospitals, the latter from Bellevue. In addition, the baseline questionnaires disclosed that very few were even familiar with the New York Hospital. There was therefore some concern about this problem.

"Feasibility" begs as many questions as it answers. What level of response to the invitation would establish the complete-care program as a "feasible" method of delivering medical care to the indigent? A 10 per cent response would have made little impact on the population and would have suggested that the program was reaching only a very small proportion of the known users. (According to the National Health Survey, about 70 per cent of the people in this country see a physician in any given year.) On the other hand, a 100 per cent response might have overwhelmed the clinical facilities. What, then, is the criterion?

Perhaps two levels of feasibility can be distinguished here. First, the response had to be large enough to carry out the demonstration itself: if the New York Hospital–Cornell Project was to have clinical experience with welfare patients, establish utilization patterns, measure costs, and so on, then one needed a sufficiently large group of patients with whom to gain this experience. This the Project certainly achieved. Second, was this method of delivering medical care -- inviting a segment of the population within certain geographic boundaries to attend a particular hospital -- one that could be applied on a larger, perhaps citywide, scale? This question is more complex and will be reviewed in Part III.

Response by Study Group

Two thousand five hundred and four persons were invited to the New York Hospital–Cornell Project. In the course of the ensuing two years, 1,155 of them responded to the invitation. In addition, 158 babies were born to mothers in the A and B study groups, and 58 of these were either born or subsequently seen at the New York Hospital.

It is immediately apparent (Table 24) that the method of invitation to the Project made a great deal of difference to the response. In the welfare cases whose members were given specific appointments at the time of invitation, three quarters made contact with the New York Hospital; only half of the cases left to come on demand did so. In terms of persons, 57 per cent of the A group came to the hospital, compared with only 34 per cent of the B group individuals.

This difference is particularly true of the family cases (Table 25). Single-person cases tended to come in response to both types of invitation (77 per cent versus 64 per cent). But family cases were twice as likely to respond to a specific appointment (a case-response of 70 per cent versus 37 per cent).

Table 26 presents details on the single cases and, following the welfare categorization, shows that the biggest difference between A and B groups occurred with the aged (79 per cent of the A group on Old Age Assistance versus 66 per cent of the B group) and the single unemployed (72 per cent of the A group single persons on Home Relief versus 54 per cent of the B group). The disabled patients, on Aid to the Disabled or Pending Aid to the Disabled (that is, awaiting disability evaluation to see if they qualified for this category of relief), showed little difference between A and B group (78 per cent versus 72 per cent), because those needing disability evaluation were sent appointments to the clinic for this examination. (The doctor filled out a PAD form, to be reviewed by the State Review Team.) Thus, the distinction between the A (appointment) and B (demand) groups breaks down for some of these patients. The number of B group persons examined was 75, or 6 per cent of the B group population, so that the general difference between A and B group is not seriously impaired.

More than half of all welfare cases on the Project were single-person cases, but by no means did all of them live alone. It was postulated that those who did live entirely alone might be lonelier, sicker, and readier to try the Project, but the last of these assumptions did not prove to be the case. There was no significant difference in response to the invitation between those who lived alone and those who did not.

Despite the fact that welfare clients are so often reclassified, it is useful to consider for single cases their welfare category at intake, because it does to some extent describe why a particular person needed assistance at that particular time. In the Old Age Assistance and Medical Aid to the Aged categories, age is the reason. The categories of Home Relief (with the exception of short-term Home Relief cases, for whom assistance may be one brief episode in an otherwise self-supporting life), Pending Aid to the Disabled, and Aid to the Disabled may be thought of, in general, as stages along the road to disability.

24. Response of study group to Project invitation, by method of invitation.

Group	Welfare cases invited	Cases that came for care Number	Per cent	Persons invited	Persons who came for care Number	Per cent
A (appointment)	538	396	74	1,331	760	57
B (demand)	491	249	51	1,173	395	34
Total	1,029	645	63	2,504	1,155[a]	46

[a]Two of the 1,155 who came for care left without seeing a doctor and are therefore excluded from the clinical chapters that follow.

25. Response of study group to Project invitation, by group and by single and family cases.

Group	Welfare cases	Cases that came Number	Per cent	Persons	Persons who came Number	Per cent
A (appointment)						
Single cases	277	213	77	277	213	77
Family cases	261	183	70	1,054	547	52
Total	538	396	74	1,331	760	52
B (demand)						
Single cases	256	163	64	256	163	64
Family cases	235	86	37	917	232	25
Total	491	249	51	1,173	395	34
A + B						
Single cases	533	376	71	533	376	71
Family cases	496	269	54	1,971	779	40
Total	1,029	645	63	2,504	1,155	46

26. Response of single cases to Project invitation, by study group and welfare category.

Group	Total cases	Cases that came	
		Number	Per cent
A (appointment)			
Aged (OAA, MAA)	99	78	79
Disabled (AD, PAD, AB)	118	92	78
Unemployed (HR)	60	43	72
Total	277	213	77
B (demand)			
Aged	71	47	66
Disabled	92	66	72
Unemployed	93	50	54
Total	256	163	64
A + B			
Aged	170	125	74
Disabled	210	158	75
Unemployed	153	93	61
Total	533	376	71

For family cases, welfare category is less useful. All these cases are on relief because of unemployment, insufficient earnings, or the total absence of a breadwinner; and practically all have dependent children. At best, the welfare category designation distinguishes the case head (for instance, an employable father would be on TADC but an unemployable father would be on ADC); it does not help particularly in the description of other family members. Family cases were therefore analyzed in terms of the age of their members; the behavior of the adults, teenagers, and children is described separately. The age breakdowns allow for the usual clinical divisions into medicine and pediatrics; the teenagers, defined as those aged 13—17 at intake, are grouped separately because they are in fact children but would be seen mainly in the adult clinics.

Table 27 shows the response of these various family case members. When both study groups are combined, there is little difference in response between the adults, teenagers, and children. The teenagers are perhaps the least likely to come. But when the two types of invitation

27. Response of family members to Project invitation, by study group and age group.

Group	Total persons	Persons who came	
		Number	Per cent
A (appointment)			
Adults 18 or over	342	179	51
Teenagers 13–17	101	42	42
Children under 13	611	330	54
Total	1,054	547	52
B (demand)			
Adults 18 or over	322	85	26
Teenagers 13–17	76	21	28
Children under 13	519	126	24
Total	917	232	25
A + B			
Adults 18 or over	664	260	39
Teenagers 13–17	177	63	36
Children under 13	1,130	456	40
Total	1,971	779	40

are compared, the invitation with a specific appointment was found to have the greatest effect on the children, or rather, on the mother's willingness to bring the children. More than one half of the A group children were brought to the New York Hospital, often for preventive care rather than treatment at the first visit; less than one fourth of the B group children ever reached the Project. Family adults were also far more likely to come when given an appointment; teenagers were least likely to be affected by the type of invitation.

Area of Residence and Ethnic Group

The Project population is extremely mobile. Over one third of the home interview respondents were found to have moved between the first and second wave interview (mostly within Manhattan), and it has not been possible to relate the date of attendance at the New York Hospital to the address at that particular time. Nevertheless, despite these limitations, Table 28 does show a relationship between intake address and response to the Project.

28. Response of study group to Project invitation, by address at intake (total study group persons).

Address	Number of persons	Persons who came	
		Number	Per cent
6th–13th Street	853	329	38
14th–29th Street	281	156	56
30th–56th Street	110	72	65
57th–95th Street[a]	316	207	66
96th–106th Street	944	391	41
Total	2,504	1,155	46

[a]New York Hospital District

The effect of area of residence on attendance or non-attendance at the New York Hospital cannot be examined, however, without a control for ethnic group. The interrelationship of these factors has been outlined in Chapter 3. Appendix Table A-12 shows that the relationship of distance from the hospital at the time of invitation and tendency to go there or not for medical care persists within each of the main ethnic groups except for the Negro group (and here the number living in the middle of the district provides too small a base to come to any firm conclusion). However, the population in areas near the hospital was predominantly non-Puerto Rican white, and this group in general, responded better than Puerto Ricans or Negroes. In other words, response was independently correlated with geographical location and with ethnic group: those most likely to come also tended to live nearer the hospital.

Permanence of the Response

So far, the analysis has only distinguished between those who did or did not attend the New York Hospital after receiving the invitation to do so. But the aim of the Project was not just to make contact with the patients: it was to make the New York Hospital their main source of medical care. The criteria of success, then, are the proportion of care rendered to each patient rather than the total amount of services and the permanence, rather than the promptness, of the response to the invitation (see Chapter 10).

The final home interview, at the end of the two year experimental period, inquired of all respondents their future plans for obtaining medical care. The interviewer asked if they and their families had somewhere they considered a "main place" to go for medical care and under what circumstances they would consider going elsewhere (or where they expected to go if they did not have a "main place"). The answers to these questions were then combined with data on the actual behavior of the people obtaining medical care during the observation period. A classification of welfare cases, rather than individuals, was evolved because the attitude questionnaires were addressed to only one respondent in each welfare case.

This classification has four main categories: those who came and intended to stay with the Project, those who came but did not intend to continue with it, those who came but could not be questioned about their intentions (these were not interviewed on the third wave), and those who did not come.

One hundred and forty-nine of the 1,029 welfare cases originally invited could not be classified for future intentions at the end of the two years. Fifty-six died, 33 moved away, and another 33 had been removed from the Project. There were a further 27 in chronic institutions who, though still technically under Project care could not reasonably be classified for future intentions. Half of these 149 cases did make contact with the Project during the two year period before coming unavailable.

Table 29 shows the final response classification of the cases whose members were, as far as could be ascertained, still available for Project care when the experimental period was over. In 563 of these cases, one or more individuals had come to the Project, and the great majority of them intended to continue with it for future care. There were 317 cases, none of whose members had come in as of the end of the study

29. Final response classification of study group cases believed still available for care at end of study period (welfare cases).

Response	Welfare cases	
	Number	Per cent
Came, intended to stay	415	47
Came, can't tell intentions	49	6
Came, did not intend to stay	99	11
Did not come	317	36
Total	880	100

period. In 41 of these, the respondent did mention the possibility of coming in the future; some did make contact for the first time in the third year after invitation.

The reliability of a respondent's statements in a home interview about where he expects to go in the future for medical care may well be questioned, and the area was explored in the second home interview as well as in the third. Table 30 compares stated intentions at the end of the first study year with actual behavior during the second year. From the results it appears that, among the cases that came in the first year, some confidence can be placed in a positive statement by the home interview respondent at the end of that time that at least some case members intend to continue to use the hospital; a negative statement is not reliable. Ninety per cent of those saying on the second wave that they would use the New York Hospital in the future did so in the following year; but nearly half of those who had attended in the past and said they did *not* intend to stay, did in fact attend the New York Hospital in the second year. Of those who had attended in the first year but could not be re-interviewed, almost half also attended in the second year. If these relationships (of close correlation between positive intentions and behavior but weak correlation between negative intentions and behavior) continue to hold, then Table 29 can be interpreted as giving a minimum estimate of the people who would stay with the Project into the third year, past the end of the experimental period.

The evidence from these tables suggests a developing sense of loyalty on the part of the patients. Any attrition that occurred was due mainly to natural causes such as death, long-term institutionalization of very sick patients, and moves away from the city.

Response within Families

One final factor bearing on the completeness of the change in utilization patterns initiated by the Project concerns the behavior *within*

30. For respondents attending the New York Hospital, comparison of stated intentions to continue or not with behavior in the second year.

Intention at end of first year	Came in second year		Did not come in second year		Total	
	Number	Per cent	Number	Per cent	Number	Per cent
To use NYH in future	333	90	38	10	371	100
Not to use NYH in future	32	47	36	53	68	100
Not interviewed on second wave	42	48	45	52	87	100
Total	407	77	119	23	526	100

family units. Once contact had been made with one member of a family, what were the prospects of bringing the other family members in if medical care was needed?

Taking account not only of those groupings of people that made up a welfare case but of the more familiar grouping of persons on the Project who lived in the same household (this is done by combining the mutual cases), the findings are that 321 adults (50 per cent of adults seen, 28 per cent of *all* the patients seen) were single adults, not related to and not living with any other Project patients: for them the question of response within families does not arise. All the 833 remaining patients were related to or living with other patients on the Project who had been invited for care, whether or not they accepted the invitation. Among them, the chances were good that if one member of a family came to the hospital, other family members would follow suit (see Appendix Table A-13).

The 833 family members who came to the Project belonged to family groups containing 1,177 persons altogether; in all the families who had any kind of contact with the Project, 71 per cent of their members did come for medical care. Adult members were slightly more likely to come for care than children. In the latter case, it was chiefly the teenagers and older school children who did not come when other family members did; many of these may not have seen a doctor during the two years. Single-parent families who came were more likely to bring all family members than were those with both parents in the household, but the difference was not great.

The way in which the clinical services at the New York Hospital were organized to care for those members of the study group who responded to the invitation are outlined below, followed by a description of medical care by the Project during the three calendar years 1961–1964, allowing for each welfare case a two year period of care and intensive study. As each patient on the Project completed his two years after intake, he continued to receive medical care from the Project in the same way through the remainder of 1963–64 and in many instances beyond that time; but collection of research data ceased as of the completion of the two years of observation, and all findings in this book will be confined to the two year experimental period.

Clinical Staff

The adult medical and pediatric units of the Project were established within the general medical and pediatric clinics of the New York Hospital. Each unit was under the direction of a full-time specialist in internal medicine or pediatrics, assisted by part-time Board-eligible or -certified physicians. Both directors spent approximately one third of their time seeing patients, the remainder of Project time being devoted to administrative duties, conferences, research, and teaching. There were four half-time physicians in the adult unit and two in pediatrics. Each physician saw patients for approximately ten three-hour sessions per month. In addition, each covered emergency calls one week a month and devoted one to two half-days each week to department duties and teaching.

The clinical staff included a psychiatrist who worked with the Project on a half-time basis. He served primarily as a consultant although he did carry a small group of patients in short-term psychotherapy.

Public Health nurses were originally assigned full-time to both the adult medicine and pediatric units, and a nursing coordinator was appointed at the supervisory level. After the first year, the Project nurse in pediatrics was needed only part-time.

Social service to Project patients was provided mainly by the case workers regularly assigned to the general medical and general pediatric clinics. However, a social service coordinator was appointed full-time to the Project staff. She was responsible for guiding and coordinating the casework given to Project patients and served as liaison between the Project staff, other units in the hospital, and the various social agencies involved with the patient, especially the Department of Welfare. A full-time case aide was assigned by the Social Service Department to assist with various administrative procedures, such as filling out requests for appliances on behalf of the welfare clients. She also acted as one of the Spanish translators for the Social Service Department and the Project staff.

In both the medical and pediatric units, the clinic desk was operated by clerks bilingual in Spanish and English; these two clerks received Project patients, administered the appointment books, kept family records current, answered telephones, and handled patient carfare payments. They also acted, when necessary, as interpreters for the non-Spanish-speaking members of the staff.

Clinical Work-up

Early in the development of the Project's clinical program, considerable thought was given to the kind of initial work-up Project doctors should do. The decision was to do a complete history and physical examination on every new patient. The initial clinical write-up, including the history and physical examination, was recorded for adult patients on a form that became part of the hospital unit record. The form used simply guaranteed adherence to the classical format for recording the history and physical, and, in addition, it speeded the recording. In the pediatric unit, a complete history was taken and patients were given a physical examination at the time of the first scheduled visit. In contrast to usage in the medical unit, no special form was used to record the findings.

It was decided not to use a multiphasic screening approach. Instead of a formal screening, care was initiated on all adult patients as soon as they came to the Project, with routine chest X-ray, serological test for syphilis, complete blood count, and urinalysis, in addition to history and physical examination, with Papanicolaou smears on every female patient. In pediatrics, a yearly urinalysis and tuberculin test were done on all patients; and hemoglobin determination and a ferric chloride test were considered routine procedures for certain age groups. Stool examination for ova and parasites was routinely done only for patients who had ever lived out of New York City.

Patient Load

During the first 26 months of clinical activity, the four internists spent a combined average of 46 doctor sessions per month seeing patients; the equivalent figure for the three pediatricians was 29.3 doctor sessions. The busiest time was the period of intake, when the doctors spent proportionately more time in patient care; toward the end of the 26 calendar months, when intake had decreased to a small number of new patients, more time was available for chart review, conferences, and research. Over this period, patient visits per session averaged 3.5 in medicine and 4.4 in pediatrics. These included "walk-in," that is, non-scheduled patients, for whom staffing had to be foreseen. They were usually patients who had problems they considered urgent and who either had no revisit appointment or had one in the too-distant future to be useful. Over this 26 month period, 823 walk-in visits were made in medicine, averaging 0.4 per session (Table 31).

31. Composition of patient load at the average clinic session.

Patients seen	Medicine	Pediatrics
New patients with appointments	0.5	0.5
Revisit patients with appointments	2.6	2.8
Walk-in patients	0.4	1.1
Total	3.5	4.4

In pediatrics, "walk-ins" were handled in a different way from the medical clinic system and in the same manner as the non-Project patients. All children without appointments were screened by a pediatrician at entrance to the clinic. If they were suffering from an acute condition that needed immediate medical attention, they were referred to the pediatric isolation unit where they were identified as Project patients and seen by Project staff. Children with conditions considered non-acute were referred to the Project office. There they were given appointments to return to the pediatric clinic in the future, if necessary; school and other forms were filled out on the spot and needed prescription refills were given by one of the Project physicians. Only "walk-ins" seen by a physician were counted as clinic visits. Despite this, far more unscheduled visits were recorded for children than for adults.

A significant incidence of broken appointments was encountered. Indeed, an average of 1.4 appointments per session (0.5 new and 0.9 return visit appointments) were broken in the medical clinic. This represents a broken appointment rate of 22 to 27 per cent, a figure similar to that observed in the remainder of the general medical clinic of the hospital. It must be remembered, however, that Project appointments were sent to the entire A group, some of whom chose not to respond. The general medical clinic rate applies to patients already attending the hospital.

The data on broken appointments in the pediatric unit were not precisely comparable, but the rate was estimated to be somewhat higher than in the medical unit. In the entire study group the average number of broken appointments per patient during the first year after invitation was 1.7 in pediatrics, compared to 1.2 in medicine. The impact of broken appointments was apt to be felt especially in pediatrics, where a whole family might fail to appear as scheduled. The patient load per clinic session in pediatrics was therefore particularly irregular, ranging from no patients at all to an extremely crowded clinic.

Communication

Every effort was made to deal with families as units. Measures were taken to assure regular direct communication between the physically separate medical and pediatric services. Direct-line telephone connections were established, and written forms, exchanged daily, indicated the day's visits (including the broken appointments), the name of the doctor who saw the patient, and the disposition of each case. Thus, each unit was kept informed of the daily activities of the other.

To make services of the Project more available to the patients out in the community, specific measures were taken: a direct outside telephone line was set up at the Project desk by-passing the hospital switchboard; and patients were informed that immediate reimbursement would be made for carfare to and from the hospital for both routine and emergency visits.

At night and on weekends, the Project physicians received emergency calls through the direct Project telephone line monitored by a commercial answering service. The internist or pediatrician "on call" spoke with the patients, offered advice, and made home visits when necessary. When it was clear that the patient would be better served in the emergency room, he was instructed to come directly there, or an ambulance was dispatched. This approach was usually readily accepted, because patients were accustomed to using this medical care facility. Night and weekend phone requests were infrequent: in one year there were 62 such calls.

Nursing

In the beginning the staff nurses assigned to the Project spent most of their time in direct patient service. However, as time went on, every effort was made to integrate the Project's nursing activities into those of the non-Project general medical and pediatric clinics. Finally, routine nursing care was given by the regular medical or pediatric clinic nursing staff. The part-time nurse in pediatrics, then, spent her time in health instruction, nursing interviews, and certain research duties. The full-time nurse in the medical unit devoted her time to problem patients and to the nursing research aspects of the Project.

The nursing coordinator supervised the activities of the Project nurses and clerical staff and, most important, tried to coordinate the activities of the physicians in the care of families. These tasks involved, among other things, keeping physicians informed when their patients were admitted to or discharged from the wards of the New York Hospital or used the emergency room there; it also involved liaison with patients in nursing homes and on home care. The nursing coordinator was responsible for introducing and interpreting the Project to the nursing staff throughout the clinics of the hospital, the Health Department Bureau of Nursing, the visiting nurse service, and the personnel of the nursing homes used by Project patients. She also acted as a liaison between the Project staff and medical personnel of other hospitals and clinics in the Health Department and elsewhere.

The role of the Project clerks, under the nurse's supervision, evolved into one of unique importance, especially in the pediatric unit where there was not a Project nurse available full-time. In both medicine and pediatrics, patients often identified the clerk as the chief representative of the Project. Therefore a knowledgeable and sympathetic person was required. The clerks as well as the nurses came to know many of the patients extremely well. The importance of this intimate knowledge of the patients by the Project staff, especially by the nurses and clerks who saw them on almost every visit to the hospital, can scarcely be emphasized too much. It was particularly brought home to the research staff when, processing the data months and sometimes years later, they could ask a question about a particular family -- the sex of a newborn baby, for instance, or the patient's ability to speak English -- and the clerk and the nurse usually knew the answer without even referring to their records.

The extra-mural agency receiving the most referrals from the Project during the two years was the visiting nurse service. Visiting nurses made a total of 718 visits to 192 Project patients during their two years of Project care. Under the New York Hospital home care program, the Project gave care to nine different patients for a total of 1,670 days of home care.

Social Service

The Social Service Department provided both case consultation and casework service for a significantly large number of Project patients. During both years of care, 331 welfare cases (51 per cent of those who made contact with the hospital) were referred to social service by physicians or other Project staff. The unit of care used by the medical social workers was usually the household, and so these 331 welfare cases were dealt with as 313 social service cases. Initially, the bulk of the referrals came from the medical clinic in relation to adult social problems. With the gradual emergence of school and behavior problems, referrals began to come from the pediatric clinic.

Social service referrals for half the Project population were analyzed in detail. In these 170 social service cases, more than half were single individuals, slightly less than half were families. The most frequent reasons for referral to social service were employment problems, followed by "facilitating" medical and psychiatric care. Nearly half were already known to another social agency besides the Department of Welfare at the time of intake; and during the two year period of study, New York Hospital social service worked with other social agencies on behalf of one third of the cases (nearly all of them involved working with the Department of Welfare as well). Like the doctors, the social workers found a marked amount of physical illness and even more psychiatric illness, which often impaired the psychosocial functioning of the patient. The most frequent activity of the social workers was intervention on behalf of clients who required support and assistance to secure a variety of special services or needed counseling about interpersonal relationships. There were comparatively few instances of intervention in relation to money grants, determination of eligibility, or premature closings. Often, the social worker's role was to help scale down the hospital's or the Welfare Department's expectation of self-support in cases where only a limited degree of self-care could be achieved.

In all, social workers judged that 85 of the 170 cases had improved by the end of the two year period; 38 had deteriorated; for 27, some conditions were better but others were worse; and the status of the remaining 22 could not be determined.

Psychiatry

Psychiatric consultations were available in the medical unit from the psychiatrist working with the Project on a part-time basis. Approximately 75 per cent of his time was spent in seeing patients referred to him by other members of the staff. Referrals were made for various services including: assistance in determining disability on psychiatric grounds in response to inquiry by the Welfare Department; advice on making appropriate referral to another agency in the community; and short-term therapy for a limited number of patients.

Perhaps the most important function of the psychiatrist in the Project – but one that consumed only 10 per cent of his time – was that of consultant to staff members, individually and in groups. The group consultations initially took the form of conferences centered around multi-problem cases. These conferences were chaired by the psychiatrist, with internal medicine, pediatrics, nursing, and social service regularly represented.

Of the 605 adults seen at the New York Hospital in the first year, the psychiatrist saw 111 (18 per cent) of them for a total of 244 visits during their first year of care. Of these, 60 patients had one visit with the psychiatrist, and 10 patients saw him five or more times. Eight other patients were seen in the psychiatric clinic of the New York Hospital for emergency consultation. Psychiatric consultations for children were available as they were in the non-Project clinics by a pediatric psychiatrist in the psychiatric clinic. In addition, a very few were seen by the Project psychiatrist.

It must be stressed that the need for psychiatric consultations is not reflected in this relatively low utilization, because 53 per cent of the adults and 17 per cent of the children seen were considered to have a psychiatric illness. Rather, it reflects the fact that more psychiatric time could have been used with this group of patients. Indeed, patients often had to be referred by Project staff to psychiatric facilities in other institutions and in the community because of the overwhelming amount of psychopathology that was found and the limited facilities at the New York Hospital.

Toward the end of the experiment, all psychiatric consultant services were provided directly by the chief of the psychiatric (Payne Whitney) out-patient department. In addition, the Payne Whitney Psychiatric Clinic provided expanded treatment facilities, so that the need for extra-mural referral for treatment of psychiatric illness was greatly reduced.

Consultations and Referrals

Project patients required services of a variety of specialists in addition to psychiatry. Some of these were available in the medical and pediatric clinics on a consultation basis; but many patients, especially the adults, received care in the individual specialty clinics.

In orthopedics and physical medicine, arrangements were made to have an orthopedic surgeon and a physiatrist available in the medical clinic one afternoon a week. The presence of these consultants was especially helpful in evaluating the degree of disability of certain welfare patients being considered for the Aid to the Disabled Welfare Program because the signature of these particular specialists was often required for the PAD (Pending Aid to the Disabled) form. Consultants from other specialties were called in to the general clinics as needed. The surgical consultant was the most frequently used, followed by the dermatologist, the gynecologist, and the urologist.

The extent to which specialty clinics were used by Project patients in the first year is summarized in Table 32. Especially notable is the high utilization of eye clinic services, which reflects the large number of patients who required refraction. Indeed, approximately 104 pairs of glasses were ordered for adults and children during their first year of care. (This figure is extrapolated from detailed analysis of the first half of the study group.) Prescriptions written for eyeglasses were filled by an optical vendor designated by the Welfare Department. When a significant number of these prescriptions had been filled, the patients were sent a notice to appear for fitting and delivery of their glasses at the hospital. This system differed from the usual Department of Welfare procedure for obtaining eyeglasses in that Project patients did not have to go to the optical vendor on their own. Thus, the hospital assumed a responsibility surrendered by the Welfare Department.

32. **Use of specialty clinics by Project patients in the first year,** (N=605 adults, 412 children[a]).

Clinic	Adults		Children		Total	
	Patients	Visits	Patients	Visits	Patients	Visits
Eye	231	512	34	60	265	572
Dental	188	337	39	49	227	386
Surgery	84	305	26	45	110	350
ENT	94	213	30	71	124	284
Dermatology	59	164	18	36	77	200
Gynecology	69	132	—	—	69	132
Obstetrics	37	135	—	—	37	135
Urology	28	84	0	0	28	84
Allergy	9	53	1	1	10	54
Vascular	19	43	—	—	19	43
Neurology	23	40	0	0	23	40
Speech and Hearing	—	—	4	18	4	18
Pediatric chest	—	—	8	17	8	17
Orthopedic	13	14	—	—	13	14
Fracture	0	0	2	4	2	4
Psychiatric	6	6	0	0	6	6
Others	85	175	4	6	89	181
Emergency	137	223	103	157	240	389
Total	—	2,436	—	464	—	2,900

[a]605 of the 684 adults attending the New York Hospital did so in the first year; 412 of the 520 children attending the New York Hospital did so in the first year.

A similar need existed for dental services. Two hundred and twenty-seven patients were referred during their first year of care to the New York Hospital dental clinic, which performs dental and oral surgery and which agreed, in addition, to provide prophylactic services to Project patients. Furthermore, many patients were referred to outside dental clinics. The percentage of dental referrals for prostheses is unknown, because all such cases were ultimately handled by the Department of Welfare dental clinic. Twenty per cent of the children were diagnosed by the pediatrician as having dental disease. The low utilization of dental services by children obviously does not reflect a lack of need for dental care, but rather the fact that many children were referred directly to outside dental clinics, such as the Guggenheim Clinic or Department of Health clinics.

Utilization Summary

Table 33 summarizes the use of ambulant services at the New York Hospital by adults and children in the first year. The adults who came to the New York Hospital during their first year after invitation (605 of the 684 who came altogether) made a total of 5,736 visits to the hospital that year and received 228 home or nursing home visits from the Project staff. (In this chapter, "adults" have been defined as patients attending the adult clinics and "children" as patients seen by pediatricians. To see how this fits in with the terminology employed in

33. Type of visit made to the New York Hospital by Project patients in the first year (N=605 adults, 412 children[a]).

Type of visit	Adult visits		Children's visits	
	Number	Per cent	Number	Per cent
Project doctor, general clinic	2,717	47	1,544	70
Other doctors, general clinic	227	4	79	3
Specialty clinic	2,213	39	307	14
Emergency room	223	4	157	8
Non-doctor visits[b]	356	6	117	5
Total	5,736	100	2,204	100

[a]605 of the 684 adults attending the New York Hospital did so in the first year; 412 of the 520 children attending the New York Hospital did so in the first year.

[b]Dietician, nurse, physiotherapist, dental hygienist. These did not include visits for tests, X-rays or social service.

Chapters 5, 9, 10, and 11, see Appendix C.) Of the 5,736 visits to the hospital, just over half were to the general medical clinic, and nearly all of these were to Project doctors. Most of the remaining visits were to specialty clinics, with a few emergency visits and a few non-doctor visits. Four hundred and twelve of the 520 children attending the New York Hospital came in the first year, for a total of 2,204 visits that year. The children needed fewer specialty services, and so their care was even more concentrated in the hands of the Project doctors. Emergency care, though still a small proportion of the total visits, played a larger role with the children than with the adults. Appendix table A-14 indicates the breakdown of visits to the general clinics in terms of the number of patients making a given number of doctor visits during their first year of care in both medicine and pediatrics. It should be pointed out that although the average number of such doctor visits per adult patient was 4.5, there were certain very high utilizers, for example, the 6 patients who made a total of 156 visits.

Aid to the Disabled Evaluations

Participation of the Project staff in evaluating welfare clients for eligibility on the Aid to Disabled program constituted a sizable quantity of administrative and professional work. Because disability evaluations had to be completed within a time limit in order to meet the requirements of the State Department of Welfare, such cases had to be given priority.

During the first year after invitation, 144 adults in the entire study group were referred for disability evaluation. In 99 cases the Project met the requests; in 16 others the evaluation was referred to another more appropriate institution such as a New York State mental hospital. In 17 instances, the requests for disability evaluation were not met by or through the services of the Project. (The remaining 12 cases were pending at the end of the year.) Inability to complete the evaluation in these cases was largely due to failure on the part of patients to keep appointments.

Chart Review and Clinical Follow-up

Chart review and clinical follow-up required considerable thought and effort on the part of the Project staff. Several methods were tried in an effort to handle this most effectively. In pediatrics, chart review was accomplished daily at the end of each clinic session by the regular pediatric out-patient department staff. Under the stimulus of the social service coordinator and pediatric staff members and with the support of the Project psychiatrist, weekly "family" conferences were evolved.

They provided a forum for discussion, by all disciplines, of families presenting complex medical and psychosocial problems. These conferences contributed greatly to the effective delivery of comprehensive care.

Medical care of good quality depends in part on regular complete review of charts to uncover any problems in clinical management and follow-up. Such a review could also contribute to research by providing a systematic clinical picture of the patients. It was therefore determined to fit this activity into the experimental timetable of the Project and to review each patient's chart as soon as he had completed the first and second year after invitation to the Project. Members of the clinical disciplines -- medicine, pediatrics, nursing, and social service -- discussed individually and together what information should be systematically collected. Forms were designed and specifications written to insure uniformity.

The first annual review began with a detailed utilization survey of each clinical record by the research unit. Chart review by a representative of each clinical discipline involved in the care of the patient followed, and the appropriate forms were completed. Next, each case was briefly presented at a conference attended by the entire clinical staff. At these interdisciplinary meetings, information, questions, recommendations, and speculations concerning the individual patients and families were shared. These could frequently be translated into direct measures that might facilitate care of the patient and provide resolutions for action. The meetings also served as a forum for the discussion of generic problems encountered in the care of an indigent population. They further provided a direct method of familiarizing the entire staff with the problems of all the Project patients.

Among recommendations arising out of the annual review were that the patient be sent an appointment for a special clinic test or revisit appointment or -- and these were the most troublesome cases -- a wide variety of maneuvers to return to clinical care patients "lost to follow-up." This latter group was of such interest and significance that a series of staff conferences was organized for their particular consideration. From these meetings evolved the policy that every adult patient who broke an appointment would routinely be given a total of three consecutive appointments. (In pediatrics, however, this policy was not adopted. Instead, it was considered more significant to review the utilization and broken appointment record of the family as a whole and, depending on this, decisions were made on an individual basis.) If the patient broke all three, the physician in charge of the case decided whether or not the matter should be pursued further. If it seemed important to keep the patients under care, the Department of Welfare was consulted about the status of the case, the most recently recorded address, and so on. If this inquiry failed to produce a "lead," then, in a few cases, a home visit was made by a member of the Project staff, the welfare investigator, or the visiting nurse service, whichever seemed most appropriate. These efforts frequently failed to produce any trace of the patient, and in such instances the issue had to be dropped. In other cases, it was found that the patient had gone elsewhere for medical care or had been hospitalized for some urgent condition (frequently psychiatric). In still other cases, it was found that the patient was no longer on welfare and therefore might well have believed that Project medical care was no longer available. Because this was not so, a second invitation to the Project was sent to each welfare case originally invited during the second year. A brochure was included detailing again the services offered by the Project.

At the anniversary marking the end of the second year after intake, the clinical record of each Project patient was reviewed again. This review was similar to the first in objective but differed somewhat in format and type of information collected. It will be described in Chapter 8, which presents data yielded by the second review.

Rate of Intake and Attrition

Figures 2 and 3 show, for each patient coming in the first twelve months, the interval between his receipt of the invitation and his first subsequent visit to the New York Hospital (or, in rare instances, his first contact with the Project at home or in a nursing home). The great majority came first to the general medical or general pediatric clinics. A few were seen elsewhere in the hospital first (usually in the emergency room) and then referred to the Project. A very small number were already under active care in one of the clinics and either continued there or were switched to a Project physician. The graphs show the interval before the first visit: some patients, especially in the A group, broke one or more appointments before they first came.

These figures make it clear that intake of adults was more rapid than that of children. The appointments for A group patients could be conveniently spaced within the first two months a patient came on the Project. But B group patients, invited to come when they felt the need, responded in large numbers in their very first month after invitation. The combination of A and B groups led to a high peak of new adult patients throughout the first year, although a few new patients continued to come throughout, and beyond, the experimental period. One important reason for the heavy early load in the general medical clinic was the disability evaluation of those on Pending Aid to the Disabled. Because all study group patients needing this evaluation were referred by the Welfare Department to the Project, whether or not they had

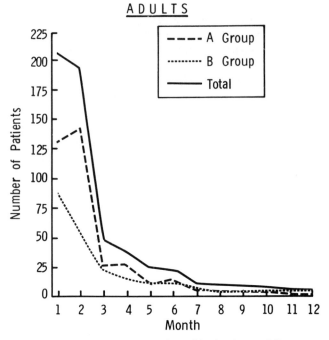

Fig. 2. Interval between receipt of invitation and first
visit to New York Hospital

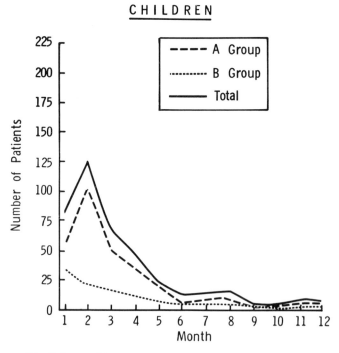

Fig. 3. Interval between receipt of invitation and first
visit to New York Hospital

come spontaneously, there were many B group as well as A group patients seen very soon after intake.

In pediatrics (Figure 3), the patient load built up more slowly, with a peak about two months after invitation for each patient rather than in the first month. Intake dropped less sharply in pediatrics than in medicine, however, and a number of children came for the first time in the second year. The letter of re-invitation sent in the second year was especially likely to bring in new family cases.

The total number of patients considered by the clinical staff to be under active care at the end of the Project has had to be estimated. A precise answer to this question is not possible, because of the difficulty in defining "active care" in a way that is acceptable to both the patient and the doctor. For example, it is recognized that a given individual may consider himself to be under the care of a given physician, even though he is only seen at six to twelve month intervals. The doctor, in such a relationship, may or may not agree with the patient. However, in spite of these recognized difficulties, an attempt was made to estimate the "clinical activity status" of the adults who came to the New York Hospital. (The estimate was not extended to the children, because all pediatric patients are considered potentially active, even when they have not been seen recently.) All available information on each patient was assembled and, on the basis of the reviewing nurse's decision, was assigned to one of five categories as listed in Table 34. The assignment was made twice, on the occasion of both first and second anniversary reviews.

A cross-tabulation of clinical activity status after one and two years on the Project appears in Table 34. The table shows that 421 patients (62 per cent) were considered active at the end of one year of clinical care and 327 (48 per cent) at the end of the second year. Most of them were attending the clinic; those institutionalized were either on the wards of the New York Hospital at the time of the particular annual review, or in a nursing home under the care of a Project doctor, or on Home Care, or in a long-term institution, such as a mental institution, but with the Project keeping in constant touch and ready to assume active care when the patient was discharged.

The "PRN at last visit" (see Table 34, note a) group was made up of healthy individuals who needed no further medical care at their last visit but who were, of course, free to return if a fresh medical problem arose.

Included in the "not available" group were the patients known to have died or moved out of the city and those removed from the Project for clinical reasons. Those classified as "not coming" were mostly those lost to follow-up, for some of whom several appointments had been sent in the hope of bringing them back to clinic. A few were not

34. Clinical activity status of adult patients after one and after two years of Project care and turnover of patients between the end of the first and the end of the second years.

Number of patients receiving Project care

Status	After one year		After two years	
	Number	Per cent	Number	Per cent
Active and coming	373	55	274	40
Active, institutionalized	48	7	53	8
PRN[a] at last visit	40	6	38	6
Not available	44	6	65	9
Not coming	179	26	254	37
Total	684	100	684	100

Turnover of patients between end of first and end of second year by clinical status of patient

Status after one year	Status after two years				
	Active and coming	Active, institutionalized	PRN[a] at last visit	Not available	Not coming
Active and coming	241	15	13	17	87
Active, institutionalized	2	35	1	7	3
PRN[a] at last visit	6	1	17	2	14
Not available	0	0	0	38	6
Not coming	25	2	7	1	144

followed because they informed the Project that they were obtaining care elsewhere. The status of some was not known, and they were placed in this category for want of other information.

Thus, Table 34 presents a conservative estimate of the adults who could in any way be classified as active at the end of the Project. When account is taken of the fact that it covers *all* adults who attended the Project -- including A group patients who came because they received an appointment, but would not otherwise have consulted a doctor and A or B group patients who were sent by the Welfare Department for disability evaluation – it seems a good result in terms of successful follow-up to find two thirds of them still coming one year later and nearly half of them two years later. Unpublished studies in various hospitals suggest that a far higher rate of turnover is normal in most out-patient departments. However, this group of patients, although evidently well-satisfied with the care they received, because they attended so faithfully, may well have had a greater than average need for health care. The latter assumption is borne out by the morbidity reports noted in Chapter 4.

The Project introduced four innovations in hospital-based clinic practice: (1) a departure from previous practice in the relationship between the hospital and the Department of Welfare; (2) the provision of medical care to patients in nursing homes by a hospital-based physician; (3) the adaptation of nursing practice within the hospital to meet the special needs of welfare patients; and (4) the establishment of a new system of carfare reimbursement for these patients.

New Collaboration between Hospital and Welfare Department

Methods of coordinating interdisciplinary work within the hospital were variations on already established team approaches. However, an extra-mural factor was introduced by the Project, namely, the Department of Welfare; the particular needs of these patients as welfare recipients and the specific legal requirements of the Department of Welfare had to be considered. Thus, it was necessary to look beyond the usual patient-centered focus of comprehensive care. As recipients of public assistance, Project patients received all or part of their support from the Department of Welfare. Although this support included provision for medical care, they had not previously been offered all of their care by one provider of service. This characteristic of the Project produced a need for administrative innovation.

As the Project got under way, there were the traditional exchanges of information and requests for service between hospital and welfare center. Each institution worked essentially within its own confines and area of competence. Each regarded the other as generally remote and apart, caught up in its own particular sphere of influence and authority. The district welfare center was primarily interested in obtaining clinical diagnoses and specific recommendations to effect category changes or determine rehabilitation goals. The hospital was viewed as a source of information and medical recommendations by means of letters, forms, or, in emergencies, by telephone. Hospital staff rarely met with welfare staff except for occasional case conferences. Neither hospital nor welfare center staff conceived of each other as co-workers interested in the same individuals and families to whom they had mutual commitments.

The first task of the social service coordinator was to become acquainted with welfare center staff and to look for opportunities to improve collaborative work in an atmosphere of mutual cooperation. The social service coordinator thus assumed a new role with two essential components: administration (in the community sense) and group consultation and teaching. The social service coordinator took the initiative in involving welfare centers and other community agencies in the care of certain Project families, particularly for those families with serious unmet medical and social needs, who could especially profit from coordination of community services. Examples of these were families who neglected their children's medical needs or whose family life was seriously disrupted by the psychiatric illness of a parent.

As part of her effort to improve collaboration between the hospital and the Welfare Department, the social service coordinator, aided by the assistant director of the Project, undertook screening of all letters from the two welfare centers concerned. Over a period of 18 months, it was found that the welfare centers frequently requested clinical diagnoses and recommendations. There were, however, no requests for social work evaluation or assistance with serious social problems, even in the cases—constituting two thirds of those about whom the welfare centers had inquired—who were known to.the hospital social worker. With the cooperation of the deputy commissioner of welfare ways were found for achieving closer mutual understanding. The social service coordinator was given the opportunity at the Yorkville welfare center to learn about individual case needs and agency procedures by working directly with one unit supervisor and her workers. Case management in a number of Project cases was discussed and the role of the welfare worker in cases in which illness or medical care needs played a part was outlined. This discussion helped the social service coordinator to gain a more intimate knowledge of the Welfare Department's casework needs and practices in relation to illness, medical care, and the hospital. With this experience the unit approach was abandoned so that new methods for collaborative work could be devised with each welfare center.

In 1963 a series of planning conferences was launched at both centers by the Project director and social service coordinator. Progress made within the Project and the centers was reviewed. Special emphasis was given to the observations and findings of the welfare staff and to how these could most profitably be used in providing services for their clients.

Cases chosen for discussion were Aid to Dependent Children families with serious medical and social problems of concern to either the Project or the welfare center. Clients rejected for the Aid to the Disabled category or Home Relief cases of long standing were also included.

As a result of these planning conferences, the case consultation function of the Project staff evolved with the full cooperation of the welfare centers. Regular bi-monthly case conferences were then organized at the Yorkville center. As many as possible of the welfare units with Project patients in their caseload participated in turn in these conferences. The sessions with the unit staffs were then extended as teaching demonstrations for new workers in training. The Project physician joined the final meetings of these teaching sessions and was able to give added medical interpretation. At the East End Welfare Center, a second series of teaching sessions was given for the entire supervisory staff, again using case material, but slanted toward supervisory principles and practice.

Nursing Home Care for Project Patients

In the beginning days of the Project, plans were made to care for those patients who were or would be in proprietary nursing homes during the study period. One Project physician was to care for all nursing home patients in order to provide maximum continuity of medical care. He would also see these patients in clinic when necessary. One Project nurse was assigned to supervise all nursing functions. In addition, a central office was established in the hospital as a single communication point for all Project nursing home activities. This central office, staffed by the Project nursing coordinator and associates, contained all hospital records of the nursing home patients. Communications from the nursing homes were received in the office, notations entered into the charts, and the physician notified when necessary. After 5 P.M. and on week-ends, the answering service referred nursing home calls to the Project physician "on call."

The same physician arranged both hospital admissions and discharges and, because he had a continuing relationship with the nursing home staff, it was easier to discharge patients back to the same home from which they were admitted to the hospital, when this was desirable.

Certain changes in methods of record-keeping were introduced. For instance, whenever a patient was transferred to a nursing home from the New York Hospital a photostatic copy of part of his hospital chart went with him. This copy included all laboratory and X-ray reports, as well as the usual medical and nursing notes. Thereafter, when the patient visited a New York Hospital clinic, a duplicate of the hospital record of the visit was transmitted to the nursing home for their permanent record. Conversely, whenever a medical visit was made to the nursing home, a duplicate of the medical or nursing note was placed in the hospital record. Thus, all orders were recorded in duplicate so that, at any given time, both hospital and nursing home records gave accurate information as to the medication being taken as well as a continuous medical and nursing record of the patient. All communications with the nursing homes about patients were also recorded in the chart.

All Project patients admitted to the New York Hospital were screened by the nursing coordinator or staff regarding their potential discharge to a nursing home. If in the nurse's judgment this was a possibility, both the Social Service Department and the Project physician in charge of the nursing home patients were alerted. The patient was further evaluated by those services, and a plan was evolved should nursing home referral be desirable. If the patient was sent to a nursing home, he was seen by a Project physician and told that he would be under continuous care. In addition to the photostats of the significant parts of the hospital record, medical orders and sufficient medications accompanied the patient to the nursing home where he was then seen by the attending Project physician. The administrative arrangements for the placement of the patient in a nursing home were made by the Social Service Department through the Welfare Department.

In all, 34 patients were cared for under Project auspices in the manner just described. Thirteen were already in nursing homes at the outset of the Project and the remainder were almost all (that is, 19 of the remaining 21) placed there by Project staff. Of the 34 patients, 21 were women and 13 men.

The major disease category was vascular -- 23 patients were involved, with cerebral, cardiac, and peripheral artery disease problems predominating; 16 showed evidence of mild to moderate degrees of cerebral arteriosclerosis. The second most common disease was malignancy, which affected four patients. The remaining seven patients had a variety of problems, including Parkinsonism, fractures of extremities, and arthritis; and one patient had macrocytic anemia.

The patients were classified by the Project physicians according to the kinds of services they required, in particular, according to the necessity for skilled medical or nursing services or for help with the activities of daily living. Need of these services might arise from physical or mental disability or both. Quite different types of facilities, in terms of structure and staffing, are required to serve patients who do and do not need skilled professional care. Nineteen Project patients were found to require frequent professional services (15 for principally physical reasons) and 11 of the 19 also needed almost total assistance with the activities of daily living. Of the 15 patients who did not require professional services frequently, only 4 received substantial aid with daily activities, and this was chiefly because of mental disability. Actually, 6 of the patients in this group received little professional or other help: they were largely custodial patients.

Those patients placed in the nursing homes by the Project staff required much more professional service than those who were already in the nursing homes when they became Project patients. The former group of 21 patients took up 4,326 bed days in the two year study period, and those already in homes (13 patients) took up 9,022 bed days. The latter group contained all of the custodial care patients and required much less professional service.

The nursing homes were found to be providing a wide range of services: care of the terminally ill, substantial professional service as well as assistance in daily living to the chronically ill, simple housekeeping custodial services, and the care of a significant number of patients with mental incapacity.

An attempt was also made to use the nursing home in a new way, that is, in case of acute illness or episode. Among those placed in nursing homes were two patients in the pilot group and one patient from the study group who otherwise would have been placed in a hospital. These three patients -- one with acute thrombophlebitis, one with acute asthma, and one with labile uncontrolled diabetes -- were cared for quite successfully in the nursing home. They had short stays there and were then discharged to their homes. Each of these patients had had a previous episode of the same condition but had been hospitalized on that occasion.

The study group had a larger number of patients in nursing homes than the control group (34 of the 1,194 adults in contrast to 15 out of 782), a larger proportion of men, many more hospitalizations, and a much greater mortality rate. Thus, the Project seems to have been more likely to use the nursing home for terminal care than does the existing system. In both study and control groups, those patients already in nursing homes at the inception of the Project accounted for more of the total bed occupancy than did those entering during the experimental period. It would seem that, unless early discharge or death occurs, most patients placed in nursing homes become permanent residents.

Experience on the Project indicated that major inadequacies in structure, staffing, and organization prevail in many nursing homes and that the isolation of nursing homes from the main currents of medical care is a grave problem. A particularly striking defect seems to be the failure to think of nursing homes as social environments in which large numbers of people spend many years. Providing certain physical advantages to these incapacitated people is not enough; a bed is not a home. Failure to consider the importance of the patient's environment has produced problems that have long demanded serious examination and correction. These problems are particularly acute in the case of patients with mental disability. Special attention should be given to the patient who has just been placed in a nursing home, to evaluate his prognosis, and to make the earliest possible plans to place him according to his needs. He should be discharged home as soon as possible, because the longer he remains in the home the more difficult it is likely to be to discharge him. Increased efforts should be made by both public and private agencies to integrate nursing homes as extended care facilities with the hospital and clinic system.

Changes in Nursing Practice within the Hospital

Nurses in the New York Hospital—Cornell Project did not limit themselves to the traditional role of the clinic nurse. They also applied the principles of public health nursing and preventive medicine and carried out nursing research. In her more traditional role, the nurse in the general medical clinic greeted and prepared the patient for the clinic visit. Afterwards, she discussed the doctor's recommendations and findings with the patient. She assessed the patient's readiness to carry out instructions, explained and interpreted as needed, and taught general health principles as well. In so doing, the Project nurse often learned of problems that would then be brought to the attention of the doctor or other staff member.

A new function for the nurse was to initiate referrals for dental care and podiatry, using the services of both the hospital and the Department of Welfare. She served as a liaison agent in the process of securing eye glasses and paid particular attention to patients with special problems, for example, elderly patients who had considerable difficulty adjusting to cataract lenses.

A primary responsibility of the Project nursing staff was coordinating Project services within the hospital. They were diligent in keeping the doctors, social workers, and others informed of patients' activities. The Project nurse became a coordinator between general medical, pediatric, and specialty clinics, as well as in-patient pavilions and community nursing agencies. There were a great many difficulties in attempting to coordinate the medical care of Project patients who were in nursing homes. The hospital and the nursing homes concerned had no previously established relationship, and intensive effort was necessary to insure that medical orders would be carried out in the nursing homes. The Project nurses made a number of home visits in the initial phase of the Project to help evaluate the kind of medical or nursing care that might be indicated. By and large, however, the visiting nurse service was used to help assess the patient's capacity to manage at home and return for medical care and to provide other nursing services.

The Project nurse served an important function in medical follow-up. For patients under active care at the New York Hospital, she assisted in checking the status of their clinic appointments, in-patient care, and emergency room visits. Emergency room records were checked every morning for Project patient visits, and information was gathered about what had transpired. All hospital admissions and discharges were reviewed daily and other Project members informed. Hospitalized Project patients were then visited by the physicians or nurses. In addition, the nurse reviewed all charts after hospital discharge to make sure that the patient was referred back to his New York Hospital Project physician for continued care. For those patients "lost to care," who required medical attention, information was elicited from the welfare center's files or from the workers themselves about whether or not patients were still on public assistance and what facts could be given to help locate them or bring them back to the hospital. The nurse also examined research records for information about patients who were no longer on the welfare rolls.

The nurses assisted with the annual reviews, and in addition, a nursing review form was designed and completed by Project nurses at the first annual review. This review was undertaken because it was felt that an out-patient department nurse should know as much about the patients as a public health nurse would learn from visiting the home. The form assessed the patient's living arrangements and his ability to carry out the activities of daily living, for example, physical functions such as ambulation, range of motion, sight and hearing; environmental problems such as housekeeping and eating arrangements; and activities related to medical care, such as medication and transportation to the hospital. Ability to function was assessed at intake and a year later for those patients who continued to be active in the clinic. Since the review was completed at the first anniversary date, the nurse knew the patient well by this time. This retrospective review of changes in the patients' capacity to manage personal needs and medical care gave the nurse an opportunity to determine how she could continue to assist the patients most effectively. The Project nurse also participated in the second year medical Project chart review and took responsibility, along with the physician, for determining the patients' medical care status and future medical care needs.

By far the most important contribution of the Project nurse was her continuing relationship with the patient. Fortunately, the same Project nurse remained in the general medical clinic throughout the three years of clinical observation. Not only was she in constant touch with the patients being seen by the Project doctors, but -- because her office was in the clinic area -- she saw Project patients attending other clinics when they came to the Project desk where carfare was distributed. She could thus deal without delay with such matters as lost or changed appointments, renewals of medications, or referrals elsewhere within the hospital. She was available to speak to patients on the Project phone. By her presence and availability, she became a familiar person to the patients and one to whom they could direct their questions and express their concerns. The nursing role thus became one of the focal points in the coordination and continuity of Project medical care within the hospital.

It is important that the Project nurse, unlike the traditional clinic or public health nurse, was responsible for a specific population or "practice" of patients and to a group of internists who had continuing

24-hour responsibility for this "practice." She was in a position analogous to that of the "office nurse," while maintaining standards of clinic nursing and pursuing preventive public health nursing practice.

Establishment of a New System of Carfare Reimbursement

As a result of early experience with the pilot group of Project patients, it was felt that there should be an immediately available fund for transportation costs. It is the regular policy of the Department of Welfare to provide bus or subway fare to all clients under continued medical supervision and taxi fare when so advised by the physician. (Taxis were usually used only in emergencies.) However, it made an enormous difference to the welfare recipient to receive the reimbursement in cash right away, rather than having an allowance for carfare added to his check (and because this allowance required written authorization through the hospital, there may have been cases where, for one reason or another, the allowance failed to go through). Patients altogether without money could borrow the one-way fare from a neighbor, with the certainty of being able to pay it back that night. It is the impression of the Project clerk who disbursed the money, and of the nurse, that this could be a determining factor in the patient's decision to attend clinic. Money for transportation expenses was made available through the social service department of the hospital, which in turn was reimbursed by the Department of Welfare.

A clinical evaluation of the patients who attended the New York Hospital and their medical problems may be obtained by noting medical diagnoses, by summarizing some observations about their health, physical and psychological, and by comparing these findings with those noted in other population groups. An attempt was made to discover and evaluate factors that may have influenced the pathology of the patients and the care they received in the Project. Relationships between social problems and clinical pathology were examined; factors that interfered with providing optimum care were assessed; and changes in the patients' health over the course of the study period were evaluated.

Demographic Characteristics of the Patients Seen

The 684 adults and 520 children (469 of those originally invited, plus 51 babies born during the study) who responded positively to the invitation to come for care to the New York Hospital differed from the study group as a whole in certain respects. To summarize the description in Chapter 5, the differences included: (1) *Age.* A larger proportion of older individuals were seen at the hospital; among the children, fewer adolescents were seen. (2) *Sex.* There was a slightly higher proportion of women than in the study group as a whole. (3) *Ethnic background.* There were fewer Puerto Ricans and relatively more non-Puerto-Rican whites. (4) *Welfare category.* The patients seen represented a substantially larger proportion of the Old Age Assistance, Aid to the Disabled categories, and a smaller proportion of the Aid to Dependent Children and Temporary Aid to Dependent Children groups. (5) *Family constellation.* More single individuals and couples without children, and fewer family groups, were seen. Within the family cases more single-parent families and fewer complete families were seen. (6) *Geographic location.* The group who came for care tended to live closer to the New York Hospital than those who did not come.

Adult Clinical Profile

Six hundred and eighty-four adults formed the patient load of the Project internists. Figures 4 and 5 illustrate their distribution according to age, ethnic background, and sex. There was a preponderance of women over men (60 to 40 per cent), and this was particularly striking in the age groups from 20 to 40, which included large numbers of mothers on Aid to Dependent Children. Only in the sixth decade was the sex ratio reversed. The large number of men in this age group who were sent to the New York Hospital for a disability evaluation probably explains this reversal.

Almost half of the adults who came to the Project were white, 18 per cent were Negro, and 35 per cent were Puerto Rican. The Puerto Rican population was heavily concentrated in the younger age group. Negroes also tended to be relatively younger than the white patients. Few teenagers attended the clinic, and those who did were fairly evenly divided by sex and tended to be Negro or Puerto Rican.

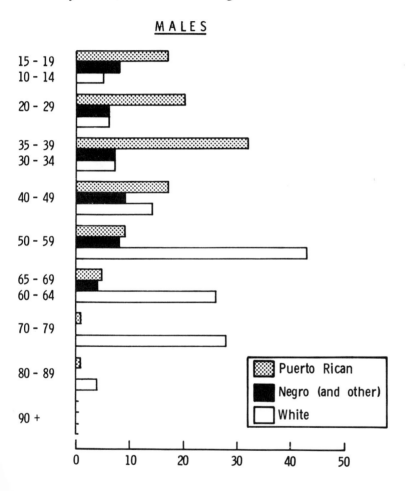

Fig. 4. Ethnic group by age and sex (males)

FEMALES

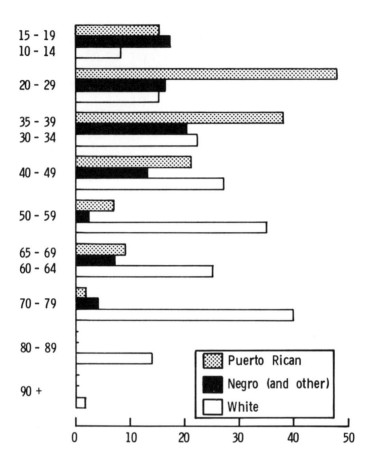

Fig. 5. Ethnic group by age and sex (females)

Table 35 shows the distribution of Project adults by welfare category. The single largest group were on Aid to Dependent Children or Temporary Aid to Dependent Children, followed by the group on Pending Aid to the Disabled or Aid to the Disabled. Patients on Old Age Assistance made up the smallest fraction of the total population of adults seen at the New York Hospital.

Methods of Clinical Evaluation

The classical tools of medical evaluation -- history, physical examination, laboratory investigation, and specialty consultation --

35. Number and per cent of adult patients seen at New York Hospital in the two years, by welfare category.

Welfare category	Number	Per cent
Aid to Dependent Children	214	40
Temporary Aid to Dependent Children	58	
Pending Aid to the Disabled	126	
Aid to the Disabled	26	23
Aid to the Blind	6	
Home Relief	130	19
Old Age Assistance	96	18
Medical Aid to the Aged	28	
Total	684	100

were used in acquiring information about the patients' health problems. Each patient in the appointment group was invited to have a complete medical examination. Each patient in the demand group was seen in the medical clinic regardless of his presenting complaint. A few patients came first to the emergency room or were first referred to a specialty clinic for an immediate problem and never returned to the general clinic; but the majority of the patients were examined extensively.

Special Methods. In addition to these standard methods of investigating medical problems, certain special approaches were taken by the Project staff in their attempts to make adequate evaluations of health and disease and to provide effective care. These approaches give a more detailed picture of health and illness than is ordinarily provided in health surveys. Among these special efforts were the intensive attempts to keep patients under care and thus provide opportunities for making diagnoses (see Chapter 6). Another source of information was the field investigation summary prepared by the Welfare Department investigator for each client at intake to welfare. By special arrangement with the Department of Welfare, this summary was made available to the Project staff at the time of the patient's first visit. In addition, weekly clinical administrative conferences, attended by representatives from medicine, pediatrics, nursing, and social service, served to assemble information about the patient's health status. Finally, the direct sources of most of the data reported here were the two annual reviews, especially the second.

The Chart Review. Reviewing patients' records in a systematic way serves a variety of functions. First and foremost, such reviews provide opportunities for the physician or other professional to assess various aspects of a patient's care and to determine the completeness of work-up, evaluation, therapy, and follow-up. It permits the physician to think about the patient, to define and try to summarize the nature of his clinical problems, and to attempt to make more precise diagnoses than may have been possible at the initial evaluation. It also encourages assessment over a period of time of the progress that has been made toward the resolution of the patient's problems. Finally, it provides a convenient method for bringing together in a concise form information that may be of research interest.

The second annual review began with a medical audit, carried out by a non-professional and subsequently checked by the physician. It continued with a pre-coded list of diagnoses that could be checked off by the physician. (The list included those diagnoses found by previous reviews to be most prevalent in these patients. Definitions broadly followed the "International Classification of Diseases and Injuries.") Another section of the review dealt with the physician's estimation of the relevance of social factors to the patient's diagnoses. Next, an evaluation was made of the patient's comparative health status over the two year period. The final section provided an opportunity for the physician to speculate about which factors, if any, had interfered with the delivery of effective medical care.

Results of the Annual Review

The Medical Audit. The medical audit was one attempt to assess the quality of care given to patients at the New York Hospital. An inventory was taken of each patient's record to determine which of the elements of the history and physical examination usually considered most important had or had not been carried out, that is, to determine whether physicians were conforming to the standards of care they had outlined. An audit was done on each of the 684 adult Project patients seen during the study period, regardless of the number of times they had come or the clinics they had attended. Table 36 lists the results of this audit. The columns indicate whether a procedure was done at the patient's very first visit to the New York Hospital after the invitation, or at a later visit during the two years, or was not done at all. "Not relevant" means that the physician did not consider that procedure appropriate for that particular patient. For example, the performance of a rectal on a patient who had had a heart attack, or a serological test for syphilis on an 80-year-old, or a pelvic examination on a minor without gynecological symptoms might be instances where a physician

36. Medical audit of New York Hospital charts of adult patients at the end of the second year (*N*=684).

Chart items	Percentage distribution				
	Done at first visit	Done at later visit	Not done	Not relevant	Information missing
History					
Present illness	85	7	1	4	3
Past history	80	8	4	5	3
Review of systems	78	8	5	5	4
Social history	79	7	5	5	4
Physical exam					
Blood pressure	78	8	5	5	4
Fundi	79	11	4	4	2
Rectal	71	11	8	6	4
Pelvic[a]	49	21	13	13	4
Weight	40	25	15	15	5
Pulse	73	14	4	4	5
	77	13	3	4	3
Laboratory					
Chest X-ray	45	40	7	5	3
Hematocrit	58	28	6	5	3
VDRL	53	28	9	5	4
Urinalysis	65	23	5	5	2
Stool guaiac	23	18	36	13	10

[a]Percentage of women.

would check "Not relevant." The column headed "Information missing" refers to the fact that this item, which may or may not have been done, was not recorded during the review.

It can be seen from the first two columns of Table 36 that the elements of the history were completed for 86 to 92 per cent of cases; the great majority were completed at the time of the first visit. Physical examination procedures represented a somewhat lower range of accomplishment, from a high of 90 per cent for blood pressure reading to a low of 65 per cent for pelvic examinations. Laboratory studies ranged from a high of 88 per cent for urinalysis to a low of 41 per cent for stool guaiac examination. The low figure for this latter determination probably represents a failure to record rather than failure to perform the examination. Stool guaiacs were frequently carried out by the physician at the end of the physical examination, and some neglected to record negative results in the chart.

The Diagnoses. Enumeration of diagnoses of the Project patients reveals that these were indeed sick people with many serious health problems. In addition to organic illness, they had a large amount of psychiatric illness.

A summary of diagnoses by system is shown in Table 37, and a complete list can be found in Appendix Table A-15. The leading

37. Summary of diagnoses of adult Project patients, by system (*N*=684).

Diagnostic system	Diagnoses	Patients
Infective and parasitic	103	93
Neoplasm	46	42
Allergic, endocrine, metabolic, and nutritional	229	184
Blood and blood-forming organs	62	60
Mental, psychoneurotic, and personality disorders	486	369
Nervous system and sense organs	418	274
Circulatory system	409	270
Respiratory system	254	182
Digestive system: excluding dental	238	164
Digestive system: dental	281	270
Genito-urinary system	244	169
Pregnancies	65	51
Skin and cellular tissue	131	113
Bones and organs of movement	205	149
Congenital malformations	16	14
Injuries	63	55
Miscellaneous	47	45

system, both in terms of total diagnoses made and of patients affected, is that of "Mental, psychoneurotic, and personality disorders." More than half the adults had one or more such diagnoses made, for a total of 486 diagnoses.

The nervous system and sense organs and the circulatory system accounted for the next largest number of diagnoses. In the former, over half the 418 diagnoses made involved the eyes; the majority of these (102) were refractive errors, but there were 47 patients with cataracts, and many with other significant eye disorders. Impaired hearing was also common, occurring in 50 patients. In the circulatory system, arteriosclerotic heart disease predominated (106 patients); other frequent diagnoses were varicose veins (72), hypertension without heart disease (65), and hypertensive cardiovascular disease (54).

The commonest single diagnosis was that of dental problems, diagnosed in 270 patients. Digestive disorders other than dental were also frequent and covered a wide range of conditions. Hernia, cirrhosis of the liver, cholelithiasis, functional gastro-intestinal complaints, and ulcer of the stomach or duodenum were the commonest diagnoses in this category.

Upper respiratory infections are commonest in the respiratory category (74 patients), followed by 49 with bronchitis and 44 with pulmonary emphysema. Under "Allergic, endocrine, metabolic, and nutritional" are 87 obese patients, 30 diabetics, 31 asthmatics, and 38 suffering from allergies. Diseases of the genito-urinary system are 104 female genital problems, 48 male genital (mainly benign prostatic hypertrophy), and 92 urinary disorders. Among diseases of the "Bones, muscles, and organs of movement" osteoarthritis predominates (74 patients). In all the 684 adult patients, only 3 were considered entirely healthy and had no diagnoses made at all.

Disease Prevalence in Project Patients Compared to Other Groups. It is hard to say whether a given rate of disease is high or low, normal or unexpected unless comparisons can be made. For a better perspective of the clinical profiles of the Project patients, their rates of diagnosed illness were compared with those of two other groups: a general urban population (of the city of Baltimore)[1] and a general medical clinic population (at the New York Hospital).[2]

The Baltimore study was chosen because it is one of the most complete studies available of illness in an urban population and because

1. Commission on Chronic Illness, *Chronic Illness in a Large City; The Baltimore Survey,* IV, *Chronic Illness in the United States* (Cambridge, Mass.: Harvard University Press, 1957).

2. *Comprehensive Medical Care and Teaching: A Report on the New York Hospital–Cornell Medical Center Program* George G. Reader and Mary E. W. Goss, eds. (Ithaca: Cornell University Press, 1967), chap. 4, "General Patient Care, Service Aspects," by Margaret Olendzki, Doris Schwartz, George Reader, and Mary Goss, p. 125.

the methods of making diagnoses -- evaluation by a physician as well as household survey -- were to some extent comparable to those used by the Project. The general medical clinic study has the advantage of having been carried out by a member of the Project staff, and therefore definitions and codes could be standardized. However, there are certain differences between the three studies, and the three populations, that make the comparison necessarily a rough one and suggest that only large differences should be considered significant.

First, there is some difference in the age distribution of the three populations, as shown in Table 38. The general medical clinic population is considerably older than the other two. The Project adults, though comparable to the Baltimore adults in the number of patients aged 15–34, contained a higher number over the age of 65 (though still lower than the general medical clinic adults in this respect). Second, the Baltimore population is the only one that represents a "population" in the sampling sense. The adults seen on the Project were a self-selected group from among the cross-section of welfare recipients originally invited, that is, they represent those who chose to accept the invitation to the New York Hospital. The general medical clinic patients were again a self-selected group of people who chose to come for care to the New York Hospital; they were accepted as out-patients and assigned to the general medical clinic. Moreover, this clinic included the syphilis and diabetes clinics, so that it contained a disproportionate number of patients with such diagnoses. Third, the Baltimore study measured prevalence of disease at one point in time, the general medical clinic survey over the period of one year, and the Project study over a two year period.

The comparison of the three studies is presented in Appendix Table A-16. For most diagnoses the rate per thousand in the Project exceeded that in the Baltimore population, and rates for many diseases equaled or

38. Age distribution and sample size of three adult populations.

Age	Project patients		Baltimore		General medical clinic	
	Number	Per cent	Number	Per cent	Number	Per cent
15-34	265	39[a]	3,219	38	118	16
35-64	291	42	4,329	52	436	57
65 or over	128	19	870	10	207	27
Total	684	100	8,418	100	761	100

[a]Includes 23 patients under 15 at intake, but seen in the adult clinic.

approached those of the somewhat older population who came to the general medical clinic because of illness. Even though more than half of the Project patients (the 415 members of the A group) had come to the clinic in response to an unsolicited appointment that had been sent irrespective of their health status, the total number of diagnoses in Project adults was 50 per cent greater than that found in the general medical clinic survey, namely, 5.0 diagnoses per Project patient in comparison to 3.3 per general medical clinic patient.

The diagnoses made in Project adults, moreover, included many serious conditions. Tuberculosis, malignant neoplasms, anemia, kidney disease, and other urinary disorders all exceeded the Baltimore and the general medical clinic rates by a wide margin. Arteriosclerotic heart disease, five times higher in the Project than in the Baltimore population, almost approached the general medical clinic rate with its far older patient group. Eye and ear disorders were many times more frequent in Project adults than in either of the other groups.

It is the psychiatric conditions, however, that show the most dramatic difference. The rate of psychosis was 106/1,000 in the Project, compared with 6/1,000 for Baltimore, and 8/1,000 for the medical clinic. Alcoholism, mental deficiency, and behavior disorders all showed much higher rates in the Project; the difference for psychoneuroses was less marked. These rates of psychiatric disease are certainly higher than those previously reported for any population group. There has been much interest in the relationship between social class and psychiatric pathology. In the much-quoted study of the population of New Haven, Hollingshead and Redlich found the highest incidence of psychiatric illness in the lowest socio-economic groups;[3] but their rate for psychosis in Class V (the lowest socio-economic group) was only 17/1,000, compared with 106/1,000 on the Project.

It is interesting that the incidence of obesity, although considerable in the Project, was lower there than in either the medical clinic or the Baltimore group. The higher rates in Baltimore (188/1,000) may possibly reflect a somewhat broader definition of the diagnosis. In the Project and the clinic, "obesity" represented the clinical impression of the physician, whereas in Baltimore all individuals who were a certain percentage over a standard ideal weight were included.

Allergies and especially asthma were common diagnoses in the Project patients. Asthma was treated in 30 patients (almost 5 per cent of the adults). The rate of 46/1,000 is more than three times as high as in the Baltimore group.

3. A. B. Hollingshead and F. C. Redlich, *Social Class and Mental Illness: A Community Study* (New York: John Wiley & Sons, Inc., 1958), p. 210.

The higher rates of diabetes and syphilis in the previous study of the medical clinic patients are explained, as already noted, by the inclusion of these sub-specialties in the general medicine clinic. The incidence of diabetes on the Project was about the same as in the Baltimore population. Syphilis rates are unfortunately not comparable because only syphilis requiring active therapy was recorded in Project patients.

Hospitalizations at the New York Hospital. Hospitalization represents another index of morbidity in a population. The rate of hospitalization at the New York Hospital in the Project adults was high. Two hundred and four adult patients were admitted 294 times in the two year period. In any given year, about 25 per cent of the adults seen in the clinic were hospitalized at the New York Hospital. The comparable figure for non-Project patients in the general medical clinic is 15 to 18 per cent. It is not known, however, what proportion of *total* hospitalizations is represented for the general medical clinic patients, because some patients may have been admitted to other hospitals. In the Project this information is available. The experience of the study group in medical care institutions throughout New York City and rates of hospitalization compared with those of other population groups are discussed in Chapter 10.

Table 39 shows the Project admissions by year and by hospital service. There were many surgical admissions in the first year; the most frequent operations were cataract removals and other eye surgery, dental extractions, setting of fractures, tonsillectomies, prostatectomies, surgery for malignancies, and cholecystectomies (see Appendix Table A-17). The impression of the clinicians was that there was a backlog of conditions needing surgical attention that had accumulated before the patients came to the Project; surgical admissions did indeed decrease markedly in the second year. Medical admissions tended to be for heart disease, pneumonia, diseases of the liver and kidney, and for a wide range of other conditions. Thirty-nine mothers were delivered at the New York Hospital, for a total of 45 confinements.

39. **Hospitalizations at the New York Hospital of adult patients by service and by year (*N*=684).**

Service	First year	Second year	Total
Medicine	46	33	79
Surgery	86	46	132
Obstetrics-gynecology	44	27	71
Emergency overnight	8	4	12
Total	184	110	294

Length of stay ranged from overnight admissions (in 14 instances) to long-term admissions of thirty days or over (32 admissions). Among the long-term admissions, malignancies and heart disease predominated, but a wide variety of diagnoses was encountered.

Social Factors and Their Relevance to Illness. The presence of a large number of social problems in a group of people on welfare is not, of course, surprising; their prevalence is emphasized by the fact that half of the families and individuals seen on the Project were referred to social service. However, the impression of the physicians that these problems were sometimes directly related to the medical conditions of the patients was not as easily documented. As part of the second annual review, Project physicians attempted to ferret out the socioeconomic circumstances they felt had a direct relationship to the diseases they encountered in the Project patients. They tried to estimate the association of medical diagnoses and social problems in five areas: family interaction, other social interaction, housing, work, and relationship to institutions. In making these judgments, physicians were asked to adhere as strictly as possible to the criterion of whether a particular social problem could be *directly* related to the medical diagnosis and to ignore problem areas that could not be thus directly related. For example, bad housing per se was to be ignored; only if the physician felt that housing could be directly related to the clinical problem for which the patient required treatment -- such as housing in a dust-ridden environment leading to aggravation of an asthmatic condition -- was it considered relevant.

The results of these questions are given in Table 40. Interpretations naturally represent the subjective impressions of the individual physicians and they are subject to considerable inter-observer variation. The results of this survey are therefore presented, not as definitive findings, but as clinical impressions that may suggest areas for further exploration.

40. Relevance of social factors to the adult patients' medical conditions (N=684).

Factor	Relevant		Not relevant		Don't know	
	Number	Per cent	Number	Per cent	Number	Per cent
Family	206	30	333	49	145	21
Work	133	19	395	58	156	23
Housing	84	12	422	62	178	26
Relation to institutions	62	9	442	65	180	26
Other social interaction	19	3	417	61	248	36

Family problems headed the list of social factors that appeared to have an influence on clinical disease. Work problems were implicated in 19 per cent of the patients, housing problems in 12 per cent, and relationships to institutions and non-family interactions were felt to be important only 9 per cent and 3 per cent of the time respectively. However, in many instances (21 to 36 per cent of the time) physicians felt they did not have enough information to make a judgment.

Patients' Health Status over a Two Year Period. The opportunity to observe the patients over a two year period prompted the staff to try to evaluate changes in health status. To what extent were patients better, worse, or unchanged from a physical and psychosocial point of view by the end of the study period? Physicians described health changes in terms of the patients' functional capabilities and social interactions rather than from a physiological viewpoint.

The results of this evaluation are shown in Table 41. Forty-one patients who came to the Project died during the two year period. Of the remainder, a slightly higher percentage improved physically than did psychosocially. The degree of deterioration, on the other hand, was about the same in both categories. Altogether, nearly a third of the patients were felt to have shown some improvement in one or both areas during the study period, while 11 per cent of the group showed some deterioration. On the basis of the present study alone, the extent to which the system of care contributed to the improvement cannot be ascertained. A number of questions can be raised. For instance, what happens to patients in similar situations under the existing system? Was the study period too short for the Project to effect marked changes in a significant fraction of the population? To what extent is the illness encountered in this population irreversible?

Factors Interfering with Care. The Project attempted to provide the setting, facilities, and staff for personalized, comprehensive medical care that would meet the health needs of this population. Physician staff members tried to analyze what factors interfered when, in their estimation, such optimum care was not being provided. Did barriers to good care arise as a result of gaps in the administrative structure within the hospital? Did they stem from the patients themselves or from the failure of the Project to "get through" to them? Or did they reflect the inadequacies of community services? This analysis is tabulated in some detail because it may provide important clues for the establishment of successful medical care programs in the future. Table 42 summarizes the factors interfering with care, and Appendix Table A-18 supplies the details.

No barriers to effective care were noted in 41 per cent of the adult patients. Where there were barriers, by far the commonest stemmed from the patients, in particular the failure of the patient to return to

41. Functional status of adult patients at the end of the study period compared with status at intake (N=643). [a]

Status	Better		Same		Worse		Cannot determine	
	Number	Per cent	Number	Per cent	Number	Per cent	Number	Per cent
Physical	164	25	192	30	50	8	237	37
Psychosocial	135	21	208	33	54	8	246	38

[a]Excludes those who died.

42. Summary of factors interfering with effective care of adult patients (*N*=684).

Factor	Number of patients[a]	Per cent of patients
No factors interfering	280	41
Patient factors	203[b]	30
Administrative defects	127	19
Professional defects	104	15
Community facilities lacking	85	13

[a]Numbers add to more than 684 because some patients had more than one kind of factor interfering with care.

[b]In 180 instances the patient failed to return to the clinic.

the clinic; this occurred with slightly more than a quarter of all the patients. Obviously, different approaches must be used in attempts to bring and keep this population under medical care, or else one must be prepared to accept the fact that certain patients will not accept being directed to a particular source of care. Some of the patients "lost to follow-up" at the New York Hospital returned to their previous source of care; others did indeed lapse from treatment altogether, and for patients such as these new methods of follow-up must be tried.

Administrative defects such as failure to send out follow-up appointments or poor coordination of care with other departments within the New York Hospital interfered with optimum care in 19 per cent of the patients. Professional shortcomings, such as inadequate study or treatment were thought to play a role among 15 per cent of the patients. Inadequate professional diagnosis and therapy were most prominent in the psychiatric area. Among the community facilities whose lack was considered to impede the delivery of ideal care, sheltered workshops were the most frequently mentioned, followed by appropriate housing for the elderly or handicapped.

Pediatric Clinical Profile

Demographic Characteristics of the Children Seen. Four hundred and sixty-nine children invited to the Project were brought to the hospital and seen in the pediatric clinic. In addition, 51 of the 158 babies born to study group mothers during the two year period received care at the New York Hospital, 36 of these infants having been born there. These 520 infants and children comprised the patient load of the Project pediatricians.

43. Distribution of children seen at the New York Hospital, by age and ethnic group.

Age at intake	Puerto Rican	Negro	White	Total
(Babies born during study)	22	20	9	51
Under 2 years at intake	45	29	17	91
2–4 years	73	33	22	128
5–11 years	121	62	34	217
12 years or over	18	7	8	33
Total	279	151	90	520

Table 43 shows the age and ethnic distribution of the children. Fifty-four per cent of the children seen in pediatrics were Puerto Rican, 29 per cent Negro, and the remaining 17 per cent white non-Puerto Ricans. This is a very different ethnic distribution from that of the adult Project patients, but it reflects the ethnic composition of the families on welfare. The age distribution was rather evenly spaced from year to year in the first decade of life, so that if the children are grouped into the clinical categories of infants, pre-school children, school children, and adolescents, the largest number fall into the category of school children, aged 5 to 11. The children were almost evenly divided by sex, with 48 per cent male and 52 per cent female; and there were no particular concentrations of either sex in any one age group.

The study of welfare children usually seen in the New York Hospital pediatric clinic (see Chapter 2, under Development of the Clinical Organization) revealed many differences compared with the Project population. This study was made prior to intake of patients to the Project; it sampled the children in families on public assistance who were attending the pediatric clinic, having been referred or brought to the hospital almost always for a specific complaint. A random sample was taken of these 656 children seen between 1958 and 1960, and the charts of 100 of them were reviewed by the pediatrician. Fifty-eight were male and 42 female (which could have been a random variation from the sex distribution of Project children); but the ethnic distribution was significantly different. Fifty-nine per cent of the regular pediatric clinic welfare children were white non-Puerto Rican, 37 per cent Negro, and only 3 per cent Puerto Rican. When first seen, almost 50 per cent were infants under 2 years of age, 19 per cent were 2-5 years, 30 per cent were school age children, and 2 per cent adolescents. Thus, the patients tended to be younger than those on the Project, and there was a preponderance of white non-Puerto Rican and Negro infants and almost no Puerto Ricans.

Methods of Clinical Evaluation. Clinical evaluation in pediatrics consisted of a complete history and physical examination and the following laboratory data: hemoglobin, white blood count, and differential; routine urinalysis (including a ferric chloride test on infants); intradermal tuberculin test; stool for ova and parasites on those who had ever been out of the United States. Hemoglobin was repeated on infants at 6 and 11 months of age, and the tuberculin test was repeated yearly. Many of the special methods of evaluation described in the adult section were also used in pediatrics. These included the intensive follow-up methods and the annual reviews.

Pediatric Audit. Table 44 shows the frequency with which the elements of the history, physical, and laboratory examination were completed in the children. The first column shows those performed at the first pediatric clinic visit (rather than at the very first hospital visit, as in the adult audit) because the children were so often seen first in pediatric isolation or emergency with a minor acute condition, in circumstances that did not make a complete evaluation appropriate at that time. The fourth column in Table 44 includes, in addition to cases that did not apply, those instances where the child never returned to the pediatric clinic for complete evaluation after his acute condition had been treated.

As part of the second annual review, the immunization status of the children was evaluated. Seventy-three per cent had received all their needed immunizations, 6 per cent were not current, and for the remaining 21 per cent the immunization status could not be determined. These were either children who were seen only once by the Project staff, or else they were school children who were immunized by the school health service and on whom specific data could not be supplied by the mother.

Medical Care Status at Intake. At the end of the two year study period the pediatrician reviewing the clinical record tried to estimate what the child's health status and his medical care situation had been at the time of intake to the Project. These judgments are necessarily subjective, especially where the diagnosis may or may not be serious. Asthma, for instance, might be classified as either "minor" or "serious" depending on the severity of the attacks. Moreover, deciding whether a child was under adequate, inadequate, or no medical care at intake often depended largely on the reliability of the parent as an historian. Of course, attempts were routinely made to secure medical records from previous treatment agencies but these efforts were not always successful. Despite these qualifications, Table 45 seems to point up a clear lack of adequate care under the existing system for children in families on public assistance.

44. Medical audit of New York Hospital charts of pediatric patients at the end of the second year (children, $N=520$).

Item	Done at first Project visit	Done at later visit	Not done	Did not apply or did not return	Information missing
History					
Present illness	94	4	—[a]	2	0
Past history	77	13	4	6	0
Personal history	78	13	3	6	0
Review of systems	79	13	3	5	—
Social history	76	13	5	6	0
Physical exam					
Height	80	12	2	6	—
Weight	81	11	2	6	0
Pulse	57	21	17	5	—
Blood pressure	25	22	29	22	2
Respiration	53	22	20	5	0
Laboratory					
Tuberculin test	49	28	12	11	—
Hemoglobin	53	31	9	7	0
Urinalysis	53	25	9	13	0

[a]Less than 1 per cent.

45. Medical care status at intake of children seen on the Project.

Status	Number	Per cent
No health problems	181	39
Minor health problems	216	46
Under adequate care	61	
Under inadequate care	64	
Not under care at all	91	
Serious health problems	66	14
Under adequate care	16	
Under inadequate care	25	
Not under care at all	25	
Unknown	6	1
Total	469[a]	100

[a]This table necessarily excludes babies born after intake.

In the judgment of the pediatricians, nearly two thirds of the children did have health problems at the time they came on the Project, and very few of them were considered to be under adequate care. In the 14 per cent of all children with serious health problems, medical care deficiencies seemed to be even greater than in those with minor problems. The 25 children who had serious problems but were receiving no care at all included 6 with primary tuberculosis and another 2 asthmatic children who had been exposed to tuberculosis, 4 with anemia, 3 with hearing loss, 3 with psychiatric disorders, 2 with inguinal hernia, and one each with seizure disorder, mental retardation, anomaly of the genito-urinary tract, and port wine stain of the face. Those with serious problems receiving only inadequate care had equally significant diagnoses, including rheumatic heart disease, malnutrition, and cerebral palsy. A complete list of the serious health problems will be found in Appendix Table A-19.

Pediatric Diagnoses Made by the Project. Nearly all the children (450 of them) did reach the pediatric clinic for a complete evaluation by a member of the Project staff. Nineteen came only once, so their evaluation was not completed. The remainder were seen only in pediatric isolation (21), the emergency room (17), or a specialty clinic (2).

Table 46 shows the diagnoses by system and Appendix Table A-20 gives the complete tabulation. Twenty-eight children (5.5 per cent) had

46. Summary of diagnoses of pediatric Project patients, by system (*N*=520).

Diagnostic system	Diagnoses	Patients
Infective and parasitic	150	124
Neoplasms	3	3
Allergic, endocrine, metabolic, and nutritional	90	73
Blood and blood-forming organs	118	106
Mental, psychoneurotic, and personality disorders	147	100
Nervous system and sense organs	116	105
Circulatory system	58	56
Respiratory system	578	309
Digestive system: dental	106	102
Digestive system: excluding dental	93	69
Genito-urinary system	37	33
Skin and cellular tissue	145	117
Bones and organs of movement	30	28
Congenital malformations	17	16
Injuries	87	75
Miscellaneous	105	99
No diagnosis (healthy)	28	28

no other diagnosis than "well child" made during the study period. The remaining 95 per cent had one or more diagnoses made during the same time. As would be expected, acute respiratory disease accounts for the greatest amount of morbidity among the children. Two hundred and ninety-eight (59 per cent) of the children reviewed had at least one episode recorded of one or another of the following conditions: acute respiratory infection; tonsillitis or pharyngitis; sinusitis, bronchitis, or otitis. The proportion with a respiratory condition rose to 87 per cent in the preschool children, whereas it was 49 per cent in the children aged 5 or over. Eighteen children had a diagnosis of pneumonia made during the study period. Most of these were treated in the out-patient department, often with the assistance of the visiting nurse service, but 5 of them were admitted to the pediatric ward.

The three systems (if dental problems are considered separately from other disorders of the digestive system) next in order of frequency of diagnosis were "Infective and parasitic disorders," "Mental, psychoneurotic, and personality disorders," and "Skin and cellular tissue disorders." Many of these were the common infectious diseases of childhood, but there was a significant incidence of tuberculosis and of parasitic disease.

Nineteen of the children seen (4 per cent) were considered to have tuberculosis. (In the pre-pilot study of 100 pediatric clinic children on welfare, 58 were given a tuberculin test. Only one was positive, and this was a known inactive case. On the Project, 450 children were tested or had been tested and 25, or 1 in 18, were positive.) Nine were diagnosed as active primary and 10 as inactive primary tuberculosis. In the 9 active cases, the diagnosis was made for the first time; 7 of the children were under 5 years of age. One of these 7 subsequently developed severe Pott's disease, despite treatment of her primary infection. Another of these 7 (a sibling of the child with Pott's disease) had the diagnosis of primary tuberculosis made elsewhere at 6 months of age. When first seen at the New York Hospital she was 11 months of age and untreated, despite efforts of the Health Department to locate the family. Besides the 19 children with a present diagnosis of tuberculosis, there were another 8 on whom a history of tuberculosis in the past was obtained. Seven of these had had primary and one miliary tuberculosis. X-rays on these 8 children were either negative or revealed evidence of healed primary tuberculosis. Tuberculin tests were positive on 3 other children, all adolescents, and these were assumed to represent tuberculin conversion, probably in the past.

Parasitic disease was diagnosed in 37 of the children seen, some of whom were infected with more than one parasite. More cases of intestinal parasites would undoubtedly have been discovered if stool examinations for ova and parasites had been part of the routine laboratory procedure. As evidence for this, there are an additional 25 children (listed under "Other blood disorder") who had an eosinophilia of 6 per cent or greater and in whom either no parasite was identified on examination of the stool or no specimen was furnished.

The "psychiatric diagnoses" listed are a mixture of diagnostic categories and symptoms rather than a systematic and consistent classification of psychiatric illness. The criteria used to affix a diagnostic label were also somewhat loosely defined; in some cases the diagnosis is an impression of one pediatrician and in some cases it is a very thoroughly verified and documented diagnosis involving the judgment of several staff members. In the case of school adjustment problems it is often on the basis of a lay report (for example, the teacher's impression of the child's behavior, learning ability, and motivation). However, it is the impression of the pediatric staff that with all these limitations, the figures given underestimate the psychiatric illness in the study pediatric population. This impression is based on the observation that, in this group of parents, psychological symptoms in their children were not often mentioned and even when specifically questioned on the subject parents would deny what subsequently became an overt problem. Unless there was a severe disruption of the child's behavior, this phase of the child's development tended to be ignored in a discussion with the doctor. This bias may also have been shared in some measure by the doctor. Pediatricians frequently place emphasis on a child's change-ability and growth potential rather than on more permanent categorization of reaction pattern. Also, because over half of the total pediatric population was Puerto Rican, a Spanish-English interpreter was frequently relied on to obtain a history from many of these parents and there is the possible loss of further information because of the lack of direct discussion.

Compared with the adults seen on the Project, the children had a similar amount of mental deficiency but far less psychoneurosis, personality disorder, or psychosis (Appendix Table A-21). Less than 1 per cent of the children fall into any of these last three individual categories.

The largest grouping of psychiatric problems occurs in two categories not appearing in the adult classification, namely, behavior disorders and school adjustment problems. The term "behavior disorder" means a disturbance in the child's manifest activity (rather than a thinking disorder, for example) and does not imply the repetition or severity of pattern that characterizes a personality disorder. The pediatrician sometimes learned of school adjustment problems from the parent or through a complaint made by the school. More often the diagnosis would be based on a written report from the school sent in response to the pediatrician's request for information about the child's learning and social behavior in school. There was a great deal of overlapping of this diagnosis with others in this area. Seventeen of the 42 children with school adjustment problems had behavior disorders as well, and 7 others were mentally deficient.

There were no particular ethnic correlations with school adjustment problems. There was, however, a significant predominance of males versus females; 30 of the 42 cases of school maladjustment (71 per cent) were males compared with 48 per cent males in the total group of children seen. Another significant finding was that 16 of the 42 cases turned out to be from 6 families.

Sixty-five of the children (13 per cent) had a diagnosis of anemia made at some time during the study period. Two of these had sickle cell anemia and the remainder had iron deficiency anemia. Most of the anemic children were in the preschool age groups, 3 years of age or less at intake. Twenty-five per cent of all the children who were under age 1 at intake or were born during the study period had anemia, and 22 per cent had it in the next age group, aged 1–3 at intake. The proportion with anemia diminished sharply in the older children. A study was made recently in which children attending child health stations in the lower and socioeconomic areas of New York City were randomly selected and evaluated for anemia.[4] The rates of anemia discovered were rather similar to those found on the Project.

Most of the diagnoses under "Nervous system and sense organs" involved the eyes. Forty-five children (9 per cent) had refractive errors and there were an additional 40 diagnoses of other eye disorders. The greatest incidence of refractive errors seen was in those children who were between the ages of 7 and 13 years at intake. In this age group, 19 per cent of the 158 children seen had refractive errors. Eight children had impaired hearing, 7 of whom were of school age. The remaining one was a 3 year old child who appeared to be mentally defective. She was found to have a previously undiagnosed profound hearing loss and was referred to the speech and hearing clinic.

Dental problems were diagnosed in 106 children, 98 of whom had dental caries. It should be stressed that these figures undoubtedly understate the prevalence of dental pathology, because dental referral was not routinely made a part of the clinical evaluation.

Two of the 5 children with inguinal hernia were infants, and 3 were between the ages of 5 and 7 years at intake. The hernia in one of the infants became incarcerated and was immediately repaired; 3 others were repaired electively, and the remaining patient was lost to follow-up despite many efforts to have him admitted for surgery. None of the 8 children with umbilical hernia were considered to need surgery, either because of the age of the patient or the size of the hernia.

There were 14 children (2.8 per cent) with congenital anomalies, 4 of them with congenital heart disease. All the other anomalies were minor, with the exception of one child who was never completely studied but who probably had an absent auditory canal in association with anomalies of the external ear and unilateral facial paralysis.

Hospitalization. Pediatric admissions to the New York Hospital in this group of children were relatively few. Forty children were admitted for a total of 46 pediatric admissions during the first year of care and 25 children had 27 admissions in the second year. Seventeen of the surgical admissions were for tonsillectomy, and the next most frequent reasons for admission were pneumonia, circumcision, and poisoning (5 admissions for each), followed by kidney disease, prematurity, hernia, and skin graft (3 admissions for each). The complete tabulation will be found in Appendix Table A-22.

Comparison with Non-Project Patients. Demographic data on the sample of non-Project pediatric clinic welfare patients has already been discussed (see above, Demographic Characteristics). When diagnoses and visit and admission rates are compared with those of the Project

4. James G. Haughton, "Nutritional Anemia of Infancy and Childhood," *American Journal of Public Health,* 53:1121-1126 (July 1963).

children, interesting differences emerge. Fourteen of the non-Project children were admitted in one year for a total of 19 admissions (a rate of 190/1,000) compared with the 46 admissions in the 430 Project children who came the first year (a rate of 107/1,000). Project children averaged 5.3 visits during the first year, but the non-Project children in their 9.3 clinic visits probably reflect the selection by the clinic of sick children. Many Project children were well and required only preventive visits.

The most striking difference in diagnosis between Project and non-Project children on welfare is that of congenital anomalies. This diagnosis was made in only 2.5 per cent of the Project children but is no less than 14 per cent of the children in the pre-pilot study.

Social Problems. The second annual review included an assessment, by the pediatricians as well as the internists, of social factors that could be *directly* related to the patient's clinical problem. Table 47 shows the results for children (paralleling Table 40 for adults). One or more social factors was considered relevant to the diagnoses of about two fifths of the children (201). Most of these were family problems, such as lack of a father, marital discord between the parents, criminality or drug addiction or alcoholism in a parent, or parental neglect. Problems relating to housing and the community (especially the schools) were implicated in a minority of cases.

Functional Status over a Two Year Period. As with the adults, the child's physical and psychosocial status over the two years was assessed to see if it had improved, deteriorated, or remained the same during this time. Obviously such judgments are subjective, but in controversial cases the pediatricians consulted each other. Results are listed in Table 48.

Two children died, one of accidental drowning and one of a sudden fatal subarachnoid hemorrhage (in a 9 year old with known sickle cell anemia). In addition, one of the newborns, a premature baby, died of

47. Relevance of social factors to the pediatric patients' medical conditions (*N*=520).

Factor	Relevant		Not relevant		Don't know	
	Number	Per cent	Number	Per cent	Number	Per cent
Family problems	152	29	277	52	100	19
Community	34	7	465	87	30	6
Housing	28	5	384	73	117	22
Work status of wage-earner	17	3	377	71	135	26
Relationship to institutions	17	3	378	71	134	26
Non-family interaction	4	1	385	72	140	27

48. Functional status of children seen at the New York Hospital at the end of two years, compared with status at intake (N=467[a]).

Functional status	Better		Same		Worse		Cannot determine	
	Number	Per cent	Number	Per cent	Number	Per cent	Number	Per cent
Physical	103	22	202	43	16	4	146	31
Psychosocial	16	3	262	56	30	6	159	35

[a]Excludes babies born after intake and those who died.

central nervous system hemorrhage. Reasons for physical retrogression were the development of new conditions during the study period (6 children) and the worsening of conditions that had existed at intake (10 children). The 10 children with medical illness that became worse during the study had one striking thing in common: all had mothers who repeatedly failed to cooperate with the pediatrician, and in 7 out of the 8 mothers involved there was psychiatric illness as well. Three of these 10 children had worsening asthma, 3 became progressively more obese, 2 had feeding problems and growth deficit of increasing magnitude, and 2 had an increasing number of minor illnesses and symptoms in a setting of chronic anxiety.

Of the 30 considered to have psychosocial retrogression during the study period, at least 23 had severe worsening behavioral or school problems. Of these, 16 were boys and 7 girls. Eight of them were considered to be disturbed children. During the study period, 4 were placed in residential treatment centers and a fifth was placed soon afterwards.

Factors Interfering with Effective Care. As part of the clinical review at the end of the study period, an assessment was made of significant factors interfering with effective care of the patient, as described in the medical profile section of this chapter. It was found that one or more conditions existed that interfered with patient care in more than half the patients (285 children, or 55 per cent). There were none in only 235 patients. Table 49 summarizes the factors interfering with care, and Appendix Table A-23 gives the details.

Any remedial conditions uncovered at the time of this and previous reviews were corrected at the time they were discovered. However, it is obvious that most of these conditions were not correctable.

49. Summary of factors interfering with effective care of pediatric patients (N=520).

Factors	Number of patients[a]	Per cent of patients
No factors interfering	235	45
Patient factors	220[b]	42
Administrative defects	67	13
Professional defects	53	10
Community facilities lacking	2	—[c]

[a]Numbers add to more than 509 because some patients had more than one factor interfering with care.

[b]In 172 instances the patient failed to return to the clinic.

[c]Less than 1 per cent.

By maintaining detailed, accurate records it has been possible fully to document utilization of services at the New York Hospital. The problem of determining costs is much more complex. Accuracy, objectivity, and specialized experience were required, and the Project engaged the accounting firm of Arthur Andersen & Co. It was their task to set a standard cost for every item of medical care that Project patients received. Basing it on actual salaries, materials, and overhead, Arthur Andersen & Co. prepared a detailed schedule of unit costs for clinic out-patient visits, hospital in-patient days, operations, examinations, and procedures. The base period used in the development of the standard cost data was January 1, 1960–June 30, 1960. Adjustments were made to certain costs reflected in the hospital records where the costs were not representative of approximately one half of the annual totals shown in the hospital statements.

Because costs of services continued to rise during the period of study, it was decided to determine the cost at the 1962–1963 midpoint of the study for more representative figures of the whole period than those the 1960 base period would provide. Accordingly, with the assistance of the Health Economics Branch of the U.S. Public Health Service, costs were updated by a formula that resulted in an increase of 6.5 per cent for out-patient and 11.5 per cent for in-patient costs.

A large part of the care of patients in the study group -- all of whom were eligible -- was *not* given at the New York Hospital because, as noted in Chapter 5, not all of them responded to the invitation. Even some of those who came received some of their medical care elsewhere. There were various reasons: previously existing patterns of medical care, greater proximity to other hospitals, and difficulties in communication. In some instances, though the Project arranged or coordinated care, the required facilities were not available at the New York Hospital, for example, chronic hospital and state psychiatric hospital facilities.

The total cost of care of study group patients during the first and second year at the New York Hospital is given below. The total utilization and cost of all care received anywhere by the study and control group are examined in Chapters 10 and 11. It should be emphasized that the cost of care received outside the New York Hospital by the study group patients is not included in the present discussion. Total cost of care given at the New York Hospital is described in terms of out-patient, in-patient, and Project staff costs.

Out-patient Services

The unit of service in the out-patient department is the clinic visit. Arthur Andersen & Co. calculated the average cost of the clinic visit in 1960 by determining the expenses attributable to the out-patient department and dividing by the number of patient visits. A unit cost of $9.64 per visit for 1962 was derived as shown in Table 50.

Table 51 presents the number of persons at risk (originally invited) in the A and B groups in the first year and shows second year figures only slightly diminished by deaths. All the others, including some who had moved away from the immediate area but were still in or near New York City and some others whose whereabouts were unknown were considered to be still "at risk" for Project care in the second year. The

50. Derivation of New York Hospital OPD visit cost for 1962 (in dollars).

Item	Amount
Clinic visit cost, 1960[a]	6.68
Drug cost, 1960[b]	0.50
Laboratory and X-ray cost, 1960[c]	1.87
Total	9.05
Updating to 1962 by 6.5 per cent[d]	0.59
Total, 1962[e]	9.64

[a]Arthur Andersen & Co. cost study.

[b]Hospital accounting department. The cost was obtained by dividing Pharmacy OPD section cost by number of clinic visits for 1960.

[c]Laboratory and X-ray procedures were determined for a 100-case Project subsample for the first and second year of care, and Arthur Andersen & Co. cost figures were applied. During the first year, average cost was $2.11 per visit, and during the second year, when fewer procedures were carried out, average cost was $1.52. A two year weighted average of $1.87 was used in all calculations.

[d]Updating was done by the Health Economics Branch of the United States Public Health Service.

[e]Physician services are omitted (except for a small proportion of house staff and full-time staff salaries included in the OPD visit total) because this time is contributed by the attending staff. Project physicians who staffed the majority of clinic visits for Project patients were salaried. This cost is included in the third part of this chapter ("Project Staff"), because it is difficult to separate from their other activities.

51. Study group persons at risk and persons who came for care, first and second year.

Group	Persons at risk	Persons who came that year	
		Number	Per cent
First year			
A	1,331	685	51
B	1,173	345	29
Total	2,504	1,030	41
Second year			
A	1,315	557	42
B	1,158	287	25
Total	2,473	844	34

second column shows the number of patients who attended the New York Hospital or were seen by Project staff, during each of the two years. It will be remembered that the first and second years of care refer not to calendar years but, for each patient, to the first and second twelve-month periods following his invitation to the Project. A total of 1,155 patients responded to the invitation. (See Table 25 in Chapter 5. Infants born during the study period are not included in this chapter.)

Utilization rates and costs incurred at the New York Hospital will be presented from the start in terms of both the population at risk (those invited) and those who came in a particular year, because of the importance of clearly distinguishing between the two bases. (The "at risk" figures are similar to an actuarial statistic because the cost of the medical care provided to persons utilizing services is divided by the total number of persons eligible for care. This method of calculating may suggest that a cost thus derived is an estimate of capitation. There are factors that qualify the use of the "at risk" figures as capitation rates, however, because a true per capita calculation is contingent upon a separation of fixed costs from variable costs.) Because less than half the persons at risk came in a particular year, there is always a wide discrepancy in these two cost figures; furthermore, the discrepancy varies markedly from one sub-group to another.

As shown in Table 52, those who came averaged 7.5 visits ($72) in the first year and 6.9 visits ($67) in the second year. It is evident that once patients made contact with the New York Hospital, in the first year at least, their average number of visits did not differ markedly

52. New York Hospital out-patient visits, by study group and year.

Group	Total	Per person at risk	Per person coming that year
First year			
A	5,078	3.8	7.4
B	2,611	2.2	7.6
Total	7,689	3.1	7.5
Second year			
A	3,695	2.8	6.6
B	2,144	1.9	7.5
Total	5,839	2.4	6.9

from A group to B group. Because of the considerable difference in response, however, A group visits *per person at risk* are much higher than B group visits per person at risk, namely, 3.8 in comparison with 2.2 in the first year. In the second year, A group patients who came made fewer visits than B group (6.6 in comparison with 7.5 visits), because so many had had a complete evaluation carried out during the first year. B group patients, many of whom came in on demand for the first time in the second year, averaged as many visits during the second year as in the first year. Not enough had received a complete evaluation in the first year to show an overall decline in utilization. This assumption is borne out by the fact that the disabled in B group, who were mainly compelled to come in the first year, had *fewer* visits in the second year, whereas families in B group, who were especially apt to come in later, averaged *more* visits in the second year. The overall decline from 7,689 visits in the first year to 5,839 in the second, however, owed more to the decrease in number of patients served than to the decline in average visits; those who came continued to need a great deal of medical care. Indeed, in each year and for each study group, visits at the New York Hospital alone for those who *did* come averaged more than the national figure for doctor visits in the general population (about 5 visits per person[1]), and this does not include additional visits made by some of these patients to other facilities.

1. *U.S. National Health Survey: Volume of Physician Visits, United States, July 1957–June 1959*, U.S. Department of Health, Education, and Welfare, Public Health Service Publication no. 584-B19, August 1960, p. 1.

53. New York Hospital out-patient cost, by type of welfare case and year (in dollars).

Type	Cost for single case members	Cost for multi-person case members	Total
First year cost			
Per person coming that year	106	55	72
Per person at risk	69	19	29
Second year cost			
Per person coming that year	96	54	67
Per person at risk	49	16	23

In general, as Table 53 illustrates, there was a considerable and consistent difference in utilization, and therefore in cost, between single welfare cases and the members of multi-person cases. Expressed in terms of cost per person coming that year, single case costs were almost twice as great as family members. It must be remembered that single welfare cases are usually on public assistance because of old age or disability. If there is disability in a member of a family, the person with the disability becomes a "single" welfare case. Members of multi-person welfare cases, then, are mostly healthy people on welfare for other reasons, such as dependent children: it is not surprising that their medical care costs less.

If costs are spread over all the people at risk (the lower lines in Table 53), the difference between single and family case members is even larger: single cases are three to four times costlier per person at risk. This bigger difference reflects the fact that single cases were more apt to come to the New York Hospital than were families. The detailed data on out-patient utilization rates, from which the last three tables were drawn, are presented in Appendix Tables A-24 and A-25. These also give detailed breakdowns by type of single welfare case and by broad age group of family members.

Within the single cases, disabled and single unemployed patients had fewer visits during the second year, often because their disabilities represented semi-acute problems at the time of coming on welfare. Applicants for the Aid to Disabled category required medical evaluations, and this brought them to the Project early in the two years. Patients in the over-65 group showed the smallest decline from first to second year; in fact, in the B group, they did not decrease at all. This is probably because with increasing age their medical problems increased, and in the B group they may have started Project care later than the disabled.

Families invited by the A approach followed a pattern of decline in cost in the second year similar to the single cases, and it was associated with similar factors of response and medical care. However, the B group families showed an overall increase in cost in the second year. This increase was probably due to a continued steady influx of families making initial contact in the second year.

In-patient Services

Costs of in-patient services at the New York Hospital were determined in the following way: Arthur Andersen & Co. calculated the per diem cost of bed care for each ward service, and they costed separately each of the main surgical procedures. Laboratory and X-ray costs had already been determined when costing the out-patient department. In-patient drug costs could not be determined because utilization data for these items are not uniformly available. An estimate received from the hospital comptroller indicated that drug costs approximated $0.50 for each hospital day during this period. Data were collected for the 1960 base period and updated by the Health Economics Branch of the United States Public Health Service for 1962 by adding an 11.5 per cent increment.

In-patient utilization data collected on the Project patients who were hospitalized at the New York Hospital included length of stay, floor (service), and details of all surgical procedures performed and all laboratory tests and X-rays. Costs -- broken down by bed care, surgery, and laboratory -- were tabulated for each patient by multiplying each service by the unit cost of that item as determined by Arthur Andersen & Co. During the first year of care, 178 of the 1,030 patients receiving medical care through the Project were hospitalized at the New York Hospital. The total cost for in-patient services for all study group patients during the first year of care was $106,811. In the second year of care, during which 844 of the 2,473 eligible persons were seen by the Project, only 114 individuals required hospitalization, with a total cost of $73,413. This information is summarized in Table 54.

When the cost of in-patient care is analyzed by service, it is of interest that during the first year the cost of surgical care far exceeded that of any other service (Table 55). The cost of surgical admissions dropped to almost half by the second year. This decrease appears to be due to the backlog of "elective" and "semi-elective" surgical conditions present when these patients were admitted to welfare and became eligible for care through the Project. Most such surgical procedures were carried out during the first year of care. The cost of medical hospitalizations

54. Summary on in-patient admissions and costs for Project patients at the New York Hospital, by year.

Item	First year	Second year
Patients admitted	178	114
Admissions	221	133
Days	2,480	1,725
Average length of stay	11.2	13.0
Total in-patient cost	$106,811	$73,413

55. Cost of in-patient care for Project patients at the New York Hospital, by service and year (in dollars).

Service	First year	Second year
Surgery	48,939	27,218
Medicine	38,294	29,572
Obstetrics–Gynecology	12,179	8,755
Pediatrics	7,399	7,868
Total	106,811	73,413

decreased much less after the first year than did the cost of surgery. With an aging or chronically ill population this is not unexpected. During both years of care less than a quarter of the total cost of surgical care was attributable to the surgical procedure itself. Laboratory tests and X-rays accounted for 11 per cent of the overall cost of in-patient care during the first year, and 12 per cent during the second year (Appendix Table A-26).

From Table 54, it can be seen that though admissions decreased in number during the second year, the average length of stay increased. This greater average length of stay was attributable entirely to the members of the B (demand) group, who showed an increase from 11.8 days in the first year to 17.0 days in the second year (Appendix Tables A-27 and A-28). Group A (appointment) patients actually showed a slight decline from 10.8 to 10.5 days average stay during this time. This difference cannot be explained with certainty, but it is possible that earlier care for appointment patients eventually led to shorter hospital stays or it may be that those of the demand group who elected to come

56. Cost of in-patient care for Project patients at the New York Hospital, by study group and year (in dollars).

Group	Cost per admission	Cost per patient coming that year	Cost per person at risk
First year			
A (appointment)	452	84	43
B (demand)	527	142	42
Total	483	104	43
Second year			
A (appointment)	455	69	29
B (demand)	740	121	30
Total	552	87	30

included a higher percentage of those with more complicated illnesses. In terms of costs (Table 56), this longer stay on the part of B group patients is reflected in a somewhat higher cost per admission and a considerably higher cost per person receiving service in any particular year. But, when the costs of hospitalization at the New York Hospital are spread across the respective populations at risk, A and B groups are almost identical. Thus, the A group method of invitation had different results from the B group method with regard to out-patient and in-patient care. Out-patient utilization at the New York Hospital per person at risk was increased by the appointment mechanism (Table 52) but in-patient bed utilization was not.

Detailed information on utilization and cost of New York Hospital in-patient services, broken down by type of welfare case, is available in Appendix Tables A-27 through A-30. The following points may be noted: (1) Within the families, the cost of care for adults was much higher than for teenagers and children, though still not as high as for single adults. (2) The increased length of stay and cost of admissions in the B group in the second year was not confined to a particular welfare grouping, nor was it contributed only by a handful of patients with very long admissions. This trend was observable in every sub-group of the B group, except the children. It was most marked among the disabled.

The steep rise in the cost of in-patient care with increasing age is of considerable significance and demonstrates the massive effect on cost of the age composition of the population under consideration, as shown in

57. Cost of in-patient care for Project patients at the New York Hospital, by age.

Age at intake	Persons at risk	Per cent hospitalized	Total cost for patients who came	Cost per person at risk
First year				
Under 12	1,130	3	$ 9,672	$ 8.56
13–17	179	2	739	4.12
18–29	359	9	11,531	32.11
30–49	443	9	21,321	48.12
50–64	219	16	32,269	147.34
65 or over	174	20	31,277	179.75
Total	2,504	7	$106,809[a] ($106,811)	$ 42.66
Second year				
Under 12	1,128	2	$ 8,888	$ 7.88
13–17	179	2	1,107	6.18
18–29	358	6	6,438	17.93
30–49	435	5	14,230	32.12
50–64	209	9	19,144	87.41
65 or over	166	16	23,634	135.82
Total	2,473[b]	5	$ 73,441[a] ($73,413)	$ 29.70

[a]Sums of costs differ from Table 55 because of rounding.

[b]Only those who died in the first year have been excluded from the second year population at risk.

Table 57. The highest cost per person at risk ($179.75 in the first year for those aged 65 or over) is 43 times as great as the lowest cost per person at risk that year ($4.12) for the teenagers. However, age is directly correlated not only with cost but also with response to the Project invitation: the older the person, the likelier he was to come to the New York Hospital. Even when this factor is taken into account (Appendix Table A-31) a progression can be seen in cost per person who came that increases with increasing age; but the differences are somewhat smaller.

Although there were considerably more women in the study population, the total cost of care for men was greater (Table 58), despite the fact that women were more likely to come to the Project and in the first year were somewhat more likely to be hospitalized. The higher cost for men reflects their considerably higher cost per admission and their greater tendency to multiple admissions (Appendix Table A-32). The principal reason for these tendencies seems to be related to the circumstances of admission to welfare.

Welfare Medical Care Project Staff

At the center of the Project's concept of medical care for the study group was the idea of continuity. To provide it, a team was organized consisting of internists, pediatricians, nurses, and social workers. As previously described, it was the role of these health professionals to give care in the out-patient department and, where necessary, in the home or the emergency room. The largest portion of their time was devoted to giving direct personal care to patients. From an organizational point of view their unique service to the study group was their commitment to coordination of care. This had special meaning for a socially, economically, and often both medically and psychiatrically handicapped population. A physician was on call at all times, and all members of the study group were given a telephone number they could call with emergency or routine problems. Although they related to the Project and the New York Hospital, all patients requiring care had their "own" doctor and nurse who took a continuing interest in their overall situation. Great effort was devoted to carrying information and concern into other clinics, to the in-patient service, and to other institutions when the patient required these specialized services. Complete record-keeping and a well-organized appointment system were stressed. Time was provided to allow staff members to transmit necessary information by phone or in writing to the Welfare Department or other medical facilities in behalf of the patient. The social worker devoted much of her effort to the welfare caseworkers and supervisors. To emphasize this aspect of its function, the cost of the Project staff, rather than being

58. Cost of in-patient care for Project patients at the New York Hospital, by sex.

Group	Persons at risk	Per cent hospitalized	Total cost for patients who came	Cost per person at risk
First year				
Male	1,108	6.3	$ 56,029	$50.57
Female	1,396	7.7	50,780	26.27
			$106,809	
			(106,811)[a]	
Second year				
Male	1,090	4.9	$ 43,468	$39.88
Female	1,383	4.4	29,975	21.67
			$ 73,443	
			(73,413)[a]	

[a]Sums of costs differ from Table 55 because of rounding.

59. Yearly cost of Project staff and patient transportation (in dollars).

Item	Cost

Physician time
  Out-patient care and in-patient liaison (24 sessions a week)
  On call for dispositions and house calls (2 sessions a week equivalent)
	32,500

Nurse coordination time (including care in OPD and at home, co- ordination with in-hospital and community agencies)	10,000
Social work coordination time (within New York Hospital and in the community, especially with the Department of Welfare)	7,000
Clerical and supplies	8,500
Transportation (reimbursement to patients)[a]	6,000
Miscellaneous special services	2,000
Total	66,000

[a]In interpreting this cost, one should keep in mind the large size of the Yorkville Welfare District, and the fact that four fifths of the welfare recipients lived more than 25 blocks from the New York Hospital. A project in a hospital situated closer to its patient population could be expected to show a much lower transportation cost.

arbitrarily attributed to one area or another, is presented separately and in its entirety (Table 59).

A yearly cost of $66,000 for maintaining the Project staff and reimbursing for transportation to the hospital and clinic can be distributed over the entire population that was offered care, in which case the average cost was $26 a year per individual at risk. An alternative cost figure can be obtained by attributing the cost only to the 1,030 patients who came for care during the first year, in which case an average cost of $64 a year per patient served is obtained.[2] Because this

2. Cost analysis is currently influenced by the concept of learning curves: "A mathematical statement of the simple fact that, with each repetition, a job takes less time to complete." S. B. Smith, "The Learning Curve: Basic Purchasing Tool," *Purchasing* (1965), p. 71. Undoubtedly, as the Project progressed both patients and staff might be expected to have functioned with greater efficiency in their respective roles; costs may have declined. It was impossible to estimate the learning curve for the Project; nor is it possible to predict what it would be in a similar demonstration in the future. As experience is gained with innovations in medical care, systematic investigation may suggest how much of initial costs can be allocated to learning and to indicate when the curve may be expected to level off.

study reports the first two years of the Project, newly organized and serving a relatively small population, these staff costs must be interpreted cautiously. Services organized on a somewhat different basis, located in a different setting, or serving a population ten- or a hundred-fold greater might show considerably different costs.

Three | Comparison of the Two Systems of Care

In Part II was described what happened to the study group *within* the New York Hospital or under the supervision of the Project staff they encountered there. In Part III the behavior of the entire study group, those who did accept the invitation to obtain their medical care from the Project as well as those who did not, will be examined below, and an attempt will be made to trace all the medical care services that the members of the study group obtained during the experimental period, anywhere within New York City or even immediately outside it. (Patients were interviewed in Westchester County, Nassau County, and New Jersey. No attempt was made to follow those who returned to Puerto Rico or moved to other cities such as Chicago or Philadelphia.) It will thus be possible to see the proportion of care the Project succeeded in providing to the study group as a whole and the utilization patterns of those who used the Project in part but combined it with other sources of medical care. The impact of the Project on *total* study group with regard to medical care can then be assessed and compared with the control group under the existing system of welfare medical care. Only the total study and control group populations can be compared (or matched sub-groups within them, for example, all people on Old Age Assistance or all Puerto Rican children), because it was they who were originally selected at random for one or the other system of care. Those patients who actually attended the New York Hospital were a self-selected sub-group of the study group (A and B) and they will not be discussed in this chapter apart from the remaining members of the study group who did not come.

Definitions

In the home interviews it was discovered that respondents made use of an enormous range of health services. In addition to hospital admissions, out-patient and emergency room visits, visits to Department of Health and Department of Welfare clinics, and home visits from the welfare panel physician, they had received services from a variety of private agencies such as Catholic charities and boys' clubs; they had had X-rays and polio shots from mobile units; they had seen social workers at child guidance centers; they had visited chiropodists and spiritual healers. The problem was where, in comparing the two systems of medical care, to draw the line in defining the ingredients of "medical care." Even if, as was soon decided, the definition of ambulatory medical service was limited to a face-to-face contact with a medical doctor, there were still brief "camp physicals" for children going to summer camp, pre-employment examinations performed on job applicants by the company doctor, contacts with insurance doctors in the course of negotiating a claim, and other doctor contacts that probably should not be described as "medical care." For in-patient care too, the problem was one of defining the kind of institution that could be considered "medical."

The definition of utilization for comparison of the two medical care systems finally settled on -- and the definition is unavoidably arbitrary -- was "any type of service, involving a face-to-face contact with a doctor, which the Project sought to *provide, coordinate, affect* or *replace*." Those services that would presumably continue anyway, however comprehensive a medical service was offered to welfare clients by a single provider, were henceforth excluded from study and control group comparisons. The main exclusions from ambulant care were: school doctor; school dentist; camp doctor; company doctor; insurance doctor; Social Security doctor; compensation doctor.

For acute in-patient care there was little problem of definition. If a patient stayed overnight or longer in a general or special hospital that was not designated a chronic hospital, he was considered an in-patient admission. Psychiatric and chest divisions of acute hospitals (such as Bellevue) are included here.

For chronic care, the main exclusions which were *not* counted as medical care were: old age homes; prisons, including prison infirmaries; training schools for delinquent or disturbed adolescents; schools or custodial institutions for the mentally retarded.

In summary, the study and control group systems of medical care are compared under the following headings: (1) ambulant medical services, including visits to hospital out-patient clinic or emergency room; non-hospital clinic visits; doctor visits in home or office (private doctors and welfare panel physicians); (2) acute in-patient admissions; (3) chronic institutional care, including state mental hospitals; chronic hospitals and convalescent homes; nursing homes; hospital-based home care programs. The method of estimating use of each of these types of service is outlined below.

Methodology

When planning to measure the use of medical services in a welfare population, there originally seemed to be three possible sources of information: the welfare recipient himself; medical records; welfare records. These were the sources listed in the original proposal. However, the study of welfare records carried out in 1960 before intake to the Project began revealed that welfare records would be relatively useless as sources of utilization data. First, Project patients could be expected to be off welfare for approximately half of the experimental period.

Second, the Department of Welfare only records medical care for which the department pays, but this represents only a portion of the care received by the welfare client.

Because welfare patients in New York City have access to an enormous number of medical resources, it was clearly impossible to check the records of all of them. So, for both study and control group, primary reliance was placed on the home interview to learn what sources of medical care the client and his other case members used during the two-year experimental period. The accuracy of the responses in the home interview was to be investigated by extensive medical record-checking; the extent and manner of these investigations are described in Appendix D.

Real utilization rates are virtually impossible to obtain, and best estimates must always be used. "Doctor visits" are difficult to define, and accepted working definitions of a clinic visit, for instance, are quite arbitrary. The patient may consider it a "visit" if while filling a prescription, he speaks to his doctor in the hallway. Or the patient (or the researcher, for that matter) may not know which of the many health professionals -- dentists, psychiatrists, podiatrists, optometrists, and so on -- to include in the definition of "doctor." Hospitalizations are the easiest to document, when the records are good, but the difficulties encountered in New York City have precluded a high level of accuracy in this study; and, as already noted, the definition of "hospital" shades off into chronic hospital, nursing home, old age home, and so forth, with the result that decisions about which admissions to include must be arbitrary. Accepted definitions have been used in this report, as far as possible, but it should be kept in mind that where the patient is said to have over-reported or failed to report medical services, he may have defined them differently.

Use of Ambulant Medical Services

Study group patients received more ambulant medical care during the two years than control group patients. Those who received an appointment together with their invitation to the Project were particularly likely to receive more care in the first year (see Table 60). In fact, the extra visit of A group patients, presumably as a result of the initial appointment, shows up clearly in the first year: the A group averaged 8.1 doctor visits per person at risk compared with 7.1 visits in the B group. By the second year, the difference between A and B group has almost disappeared: the average is 5.5 compared to 5.2 visits per person at risk. It is tempting to wonder whether this difference would have disappeared altogether in a third experimental year if that had been possible or even if the A group might eventually have averaged fewer

60. Citywide comparison of study and control groups: average doctor visits per person at risk, by group and year.

Group	Number of persons	Visits per person	
		First year	Second year
A (appointment)	1,331	8.1	5.5
B (demand)	1,173	7.1	5.2
C (control)	1,685	6.5	4.5

visits per person at risk than the B group. Beginning medical care with an appointment is clearly more expensive in the short run, but there is a possibility of long-term economy if illnesses are taken care of early.

Perhaps the least expected finding in Table 60 is the decline from first to second year visits in the control group. It was expected that utilization rates on the Project would be higher in the first year; but the very substantial difference between first and second year in the control group rates was not anticipated. The likeliest explanation seems to be that a patient comes on to the welfare rolls at a time when he needs more medical services than usual -- many patients have just been discharged from a hospital, others need disability evaluations, still others go on welfare because an acute health problem arises or a chronic one deteriorates to the point of making the patient unable to work -- and this high utilization diminishes after a time as clients either become self-supporting again or settle down to a more chronic state of dependency. Furthermore, when the person is on welfare his medical care is paid for or provided by the Welfare Department. The low control (C) group rate in the second year may reflect an especially low use of medical services by the many patients going off relief or being off part of the time. It may indicate the inadequacy of health services for whose who are only marginally self-supporting. In any case, this difference from one year to the next in the C group suggests that it is very important to consider the stage of the client's welfare life history when studying welfare medical care; utilization rates may be quite different for old and new welfare cases.

The difference mentioned in Chapter 9 between members of single and family welfare cases in the use of services at the New York Hospital continues to hold with respect to their total use of medical services throughout the community (Table 61). In the study group in the first year, single case members average twice as many doctor visits as family case members; the difference in the control group is less marked, but it

61. Average doctor visits citywide per person at risk, by group by year, by single or family welfare case membership.

Group	Number of persons[a]	First year	Second year
A (appointment)			
Single case	277	13.4	9.8
Family case-member	1,054	6.7	4.5
Total	1,331	8.1	5.5
B (demand)			
Single case	256	11.3	7.5
Family case-member	917	5.9	4.6
Total	1,173	7.1	5.2
C (control)			
Single case	315	8.7	7.2
Family case-member	1,370	5.9	3.9
Total	1,685	6.5	4.5

[a]In the second year deaths diminished the population at risk slightly, to 1,315 for A group, 1,158 for B group, 1,667 for C group.

is in the same direction. Because the Project was most successful in attracting the single recipients, the additional utilization engendered in the first year occurs mainly in this section of the welfare population. Families seem to have been less affected: in the A group, half of whom did attend the New York Hospital, there is somewhat higher utilization compared with the control families; but in the B group, very few of whom responded when left to come on demand, there is no difference at all in number of visits per person at risk in the first year compared with the control group. In the second year, differences between A, B, and C groups persist in both single persons and family members, but the gaps narrow. Single persons in the B group drop to almost as low a level of utilization as the corresponding persons in the C group; those in the A group remain high.

Table 62 shows single cases and differences in the use of medical services by different kinds of welfare recipients. From the results it is apparent that in all three groups it is the disabled recipients on Aid to the Disabled or Aid to the Blind, or awaiting disability evaluation

62. Average doctor visits citywide per person at risk, by welfare category at intake, single cases.

Group	Number of persons	First year	Second year
A (appointment)			
Aged	99	12.4	8.8
Disabled	118	13.9	12.0
Unemployed	60	13.9	7.1
Total	277	13.4	9.8
B (demand)			
Aged	71	10.5	6.8
Disabled	92	13.3	8.7
Unemployed	93	10.0	7.1
Total	256	11.3	7.5
C (control)			
Aged	118	8.4	6.3
Disabled	95	10.9	8.9
Unemployed	102	7.0	6.6
Total	315	8.7	7.2

(PAD), who are the highest users of medical service. The single cases originally on Home Relief because of unemployment have utilization rates almost as high as the disabled in both A and B groups, probably because of the large number of such cases who were transferred after intake to the PAD category of welfare and referred to the Project for disability evaluation. This seems to have happened more frequently in the Project than under the existing system, if one is to judge by the relatively low utilization of single Home Relief cases in the control group. The experience of the Project clinical staff with a heavy load of PAD evaluations, only half of whom were accepted by the state review team for the category of Aid to the Disabled (see Chapter 6 under Aid to the Disabled), seems to bear out the suspicion that an extra number of PAD requests were made to the Project because of the closer than usual liaison between the local welfare center and the hospital.

Table 63 breaks down the use of medical services in multi-person welfare cases by broad age groupings -- adults aged 18 or over at intake,

63. Average doctor visits citywide per person at risk, by adults, teenagers, and children, family cases.

Group	Number of persons	First year	Second year
A (appointment)			
Adults 18 and over	342	9.1	5.4
Teenagers 13–17	101	4.3	4.0
Children under 13	611	5.7	4.0
Total	1,054	6.7	4.5
B (demand)			
Adults	322	6.8	6.0
Teenagers	76	3.1	4.6
Children	519	5.7	3.8
Total	917	5.9	4.6
C (control)			
Adults	468	6.7	4.8
Teenagers	106	6.1	4.4
Children	796	5.5	3.4
Total	1,370	5.9	3.9

teenagers 13 to 17, and children under 13. Adults tended to see a doctor more frequently than their children, and this was especially true of A group adults in the first year; they averaged 9.1 visits each. The teenagers are numerically a small group (101 in the A group, 76 in the B group, 106 in the C group); no explanation other than the unreliability of small samples comes to mind to explain a utilization rate in the 13 to 17 year olds during the first year that is higher in the control group than in either of the study groups. This is the only instance in which the control group rate exceeded that of both study groups.

The decline from first to second year is again apparent in nearly all the sub-groups shown in Table 64. The decline in the control (C) group children, whose average doctor visits in the second year drop as low as 3.4, seems to support the hypothesis that lack of finance or opportunity, rather than diminished need, accounts for much of the drop in the second year. It is understandable that family adults new to welfare might have health problems requiring more care immediately after intake than a year or two later, but it is hard to see why childrens' utilization rates under the existing system should vary to such an extent on the basis of need alone. It does seem likely that medical care is more available, in terms of both time and money, to welfare recipients than it is to people who have just gone off relief; and it seems very probable that these latter receive less medical care than they need. Even the appointment group children, more than half of whom had made contact with the Project, averaged only four visits in the second year.

It has been assumed that, where the study group utilization rates differ from those in the control group, the difference is due to the effect of the Project. Table 64 does indeed show that those members of the A and B groups who came to the Project saw a doctor far more often than study group members who did not respond to the Project invitation. In the A group, where the invitation accompanied by a clinic appointment seems to have attracted the majority of those who wanted medical care, patients who came averaged 10.8 visits in the first year and 7.6 in the second, compared with 4.1 and 2.6 respectively for those

64. Average doctor visits citywide per person at risk, by group, by single and family case-members, distinguishing those who came to the project.

	First year			Second year		
Group	Came	Didn't come	Total	Came	Didn't come	Total
A (appointment)						
Single case	15.6	6.3	13.4	10.9	5.5	9.8
Family case-members	9.0	3.9	6.7	6.6	2.3	4.5
Total	10.8	4.1	8.1	7.6	2.6	5.5
B (demand)						
Single case	14.6	5.7	11.3	9.9	4.7	7.5
Family case-members	8.0	5.1	5.9	7.6	3.6	4.6
Total	10.7	5.2	7.1	8.5	3.7	5.2
C (control)						
Single case	–	–	8.7	–	–	7.2
Family case-members	–	–	5.9	–	–	3.9
Total	–	–	6.5	–	–	4.5

who did not come. The B group invitation achieved less response in the sense that a smaller proportion of those who wanted a doctor were brought into the Project: the total utilization rates of B group members who did not come are slightly higher than those of A group members who did not come. This difference, however, is contributed entirely by the families. This is one more confirmation of the finding, noted in Chapter 5, that the kind of invitation was of crucial importance among this section of the welfare population. Single welfare cases tended to come for care anyway -- and Table 64 provides the additional evidence that those who did not come, in B group as well as A group, averaged comparatively few visits altogether. But family members were much more apt to use the Project for most of their care if sent an initial appointment.

It will be observed that in every instance the control group members averaged more visits than those of the study group who did *not* attend the Project. The implication is that the Project tended to attract the sicker members of the population it invited, and it is borne out by the finding that those who subsequently came had reported more symptoms and illnesses on the health questionnaire at intake than those who did not come.

Sources of Medical Care. Tables 60 through 64 presented the average visits per person, that is, the total number of times that the average person in the various subgroups being analyzed saw a doctor for medical care during the relevant year; but these tables gave no idea of the medical facilities being used. Table 65 presents the major sources of ambulant care according to the breakdowns listed at the beginning of this chapter, namely: hospital clinic visits, to out-patient clinic or emergency room; non-hospital clinic visits; doctor visits by or to a private physician or a welfare panel physician. Within the first category, the four most used hospitals are identified, and the remaining hospitals are divided into those under city or voluntary ownership. The second category of non-hospital clinics is subdivided into child health stations run by the Department of Health, dental clinics under various auspices (Department of Health dental clinics for children, Department of Welfare dental clinics for welfare recipients, and private clinics such as the Guggenheim), and "other" clinics, which include the Department of Welfare eye clinics, the Department of Health chest clinics, the state-run aftercare clinics for psychiatric patients, and a very small number of other miscellaneous clinics. Appendix Table A-33 expresses these visits in terms of the percentage of care rendered by each of the major sources.

Table 65 is detailed, but there seems some advantage in presenting the whole utilization picture. To make it more comprehensible, the data contained in Table 65 have been illustrated in two sets of pie diagrams

65. Average doctor visits citywide per person at risk, by group, year, and source of care.

	First year			Second year		
	Study group		Control (C)	Study group		Control (C)
Source of care	A	B		A	B	
Hospital OPD and E.R.						
New York Hospital	4.30	2.39	0.26	3.25	1.84	0.20
Mount Sinai	0.48	0.48	.69	0.20	0.40	.49
Other voluntary	.48	.47	.54	.14	.29	.55
Bellevue	.85	1.24	1.77	.60	1.04	1.14
Metropolitan	.53	0.88	1.12	.35	0.47	0.66
Other city	.09	.14	0.08	.03	.22	.11
Total	6.72	5.60	4.46	4.58	4.26	3.15
Non-hospital clinics						
Child health stations	0.14	0.38	0.34	0.10	0.14	0.18
Dental clinics	.78	.71	.93	.41	.51	.56
Other clinics	.17	.13	.17	.23	.08	.09
Total	1.09	1.22	1.44	0.73	0.74	0.83
Non-clinic care						
Private M.D.	0.21	0.20	0.30	.21	.21	.34
Welfare M.D.	.07	.04	.25	.02	.02	.19
Total	0.28	0.24	0.55	0.23	0.23	0.53
Total Visits	8.08	7.06	6.46	5.54	5.24	4.51

(Figures 6 and 7) -- showing the average numbers of visits to the various medical facilities by the A, B, and C group populations.

In Figure 6 the lowest diagram represents the existing system of welfare medical care as exemplified by the control group. Bellevue plays the largest role among the hospital clinics; in fact it is the single most-used source of medical care for this particular indigent population, providing more than a quarter of all their ambulant care. Metropolitan is next, with 17 per cent of all utilization, followed by Mount Sinai with 11 per cent. The New York Hospital provided only 4 per cent of the ambulant care to this population. Visits to non-hospital dental

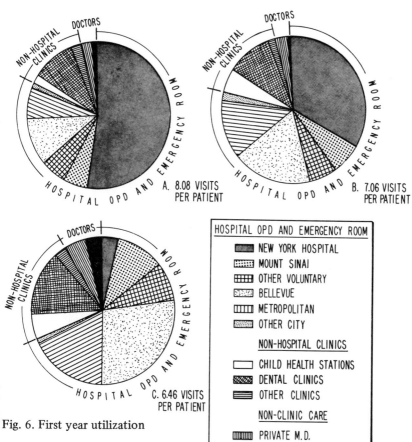

Fig. 6. First year utilization

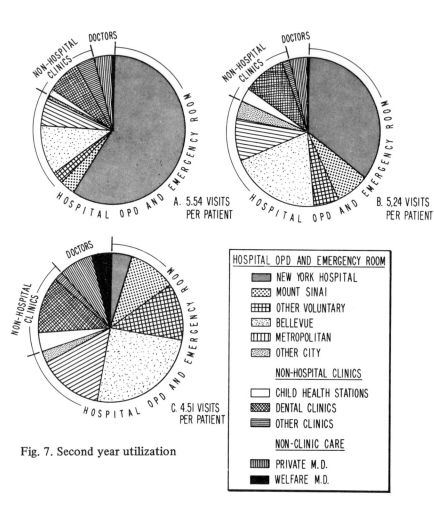

Fig. 7. Second year utilization

clinics account for 14 per cent of the visits altogether, with no type of dental clinic contributing a large amount. The proportionately small contribution of the welfare panel physician to the welfare medical care system is particularly striking. He undoubtedly plays a larger role with old welfare cases (who have had time to learn of and become accustomed to the availability of home visits) than with new admissions to welfare, half of whom had never been on welfare before. The fact that the participants in the Project spent about half the experimental period off welfare probably accounts for much of the use of private doctors in the control group.

In the lowest circle in Figure 7, the utilization picture in the control group in the second year remains remarkably constant, but there is less of everything. There is some increase in the use of other city and voluntary hospitals, probably because of an increasing number of moves to other parts of the city. These moves seem more apt to decrease visits to Bellevue and Metropolitan, whose districting rules discourage out-of-district patients, than to the New York Hospital and Mount Sinai. Visits to private doctors increase somewhat. But in general, the pattern of care does not seem to vary significantly from one year to the next, only the amount. The decline from 6.5 to 4.5 visits per person at risk represents a decline of 31 per cent, only part of which can be attributed to less complete reporting in the second year.

After this brief sketch of the existing medical care system, attention will be focused on the impact on this system of the letter of invitation to the New York Hospital. The difference made by enclosing a clinic appointment with the invitation is illustrated by the difference in shading of the top lefthand and top righthand circles, representing respectively the A and B group systems of care. In the first year (Figure 6), the proportion of care directly rendered by the New York Hospital was increased from the 4 per cent under the existing system to 53 per cent in the A (appointment) group and 34 per cent in the B (demand) group. In addition, some visits to dental, chest, and aftercare clinics were made on referral by the Project or in close liaison with it; an estimated 5 to 7 per cent of all visits might be so classified, raising the percentage to about 60 for A group and 39 for B group. Thus, the A (appointment) approach was half again as successful as the B (demand) approach in concentrating in one place the medical services rendered to a section of the community.

In the second year the proportion of care rendered directly by the New York Hospital to the study group actually increased, especially in the A group; it rose from 53 to 59 per cent for A and from 34 to 35 per cent for B. Again, this figure could be increased if referrals to outside clinics were added. This increase in the A group did not seem to deplete any one particular source of care outside the Project; there was less use of most of the alternative sources of care in the second year than in the first, suggesting that coordination is not achieved all at once but may come about gradually as patients become familiar with the range of services available to them from a central source of care; and as favorable word about this formerly unfamiliar source spreads in the community.

If the sources of care used by the B and C groups in the first year are compared, it appears that the B form of invitation (that is, one not accompanied by an initial appointment and leaving it up to the patient to establish contact) drew patients to the New York Hospital rather evenly from all the various alternative sources. There are fewer B than C group visits to every alternative facility except child health stations and city hospitals other than Bellevue and Metropolitan. Private and welfare doctors visits are particularly likely to be lower in B than in C. But in the second year, visits to Bellevue are almost as high in the B group as in the C group. It may be that most of the B group patients who tried the Project but did not stay with it were former Bellevue patients who eventually returned to Bellevue for their care.

To see how a clinic appointment enclosed with the original invitation affected patients' sources of care, A and C groups must be compared. The appointment approach apparently had a considerably greater tendency than the demand approach to attract patients away from the two local city hospitals. Considering the difference in family response between A and B groups, it would seem that these are the families who were diverted from their customary use of city hospitals only by the appointment approach. The diversion seems to be lasting, because almost the same small number used Bellevue and Metropolitan in the second year.

Welfare panel physicians, used very little by either A or B group in the first year, are hardly used at all by them in the second year, although there are a limited number of panel physicians' visits in the control group persisting into the second year.

Utilization Patterns of Those Who Came to the Project. Appendix A-33 shows that the New York Hospital provided 53 per cent of all the care received by the whole A group in the first year and 34 per cent of all care for the B group and that in the second year these percentages increased to 59 and 35 respectively. The question then arises: how much of the medical care received outside the Project could be attributed to those who did not come to the New York Hospital at all, and how much to those who did come? Did many of the patients attending the Project use other medical facilities either before, during, or after their period of active care with the Project?[1]

1. Even in the Family Health Maintenance Demonstration at Montefiore Hospital, patients sought care outside the intensive preventive system of care offered to them. Eliot Freidson has described this in his book *Patients' Views of Medical Practice* (Russell Sage Foundation, 1961) pp. 112-115.

66. Utilization patterns of members of the study group who came to the project at some time during the two years.

	Percentage distribution			
	First year		Second year	
Source of treatment	A (N=760)	B (N=395)	A (N=760)	B (N=395)
New York Hospital	69	66	75	68
Mount Sinai	2	3	1	3
Other voluntary hospital	6	4	2	3
Bellevue	5	6	6	11
Metropolitan	4	7	4	4
Other city hospital	—	—	1	2
Child health station	1	1	1	—
Dental clinic	9	9	3	4
Other clinic	2	1	3	1
Private M.D.	1	2	4	4
Welfare M.D., Project	—	1	—	—
Welfare M.D. other	1	—	—	—
Total	100	100	100	100

Table 66 shows the utilization patterns of those members of the study groups who came to the Project at some time during the two year period. It shows that in the whole study group (A and B), Project patients who accepted the invitation to the New York Hospital received very little ambulant care elsewhere. Most dental care for those who came was through referral from the Project and much "other clinic" care (in Welfare eye clinic, Department of Health chest clinic, or state aftercare) was referred or coordinated by the Project, so that A group patients who came received four fifths of their care by or through the Project, and the B group was not far behind. Even among the patients who did come, however, some difference between appointment and demand approaches persists. The tendency for the A group in the second year was for their ambulant care to become even more centered at the New York Hospital (75 per cent of all care given); but in the B group the counter-attraction of Bellevue seems to have persuaded some patients to go back to it from the New York Hospital.

It was not possible to document the chronology of events for all Project patients who used other sources of care besides the New York

Hospital, because so much detail could not reliably be obtained from the home interviews. But records were checked in the 100-case study group sub-sample for dates of clinic attendance at the various hospitals. Some patients attended other clinics before coming to the Project; several of these were high utilizers of medical service who were finally required by the Welfare Department to undergo PAD evaluation at the New York Hospital. Several others tried the Project but returned to their previous sources of care. Practically none seems to have attended the New York Hospital and other hospital clinics simultaneously and for the same condition. In this small group carefully investigated, "clinic shopping" and duplication seem to have been virtually eliminated.

The Use of In-patient Services

In addition to receiving more ambulant medical care, members of the study group received more in-patient care than those in the control group. In Table 67 the admissions to general hospitals are presented, and rates in the A, B, and C groups are compared against the background of the rates for the whole nation.

These figures represent a best estimate of the hospitalization rates in the three groups. Details of the method used in arriving at the estimates can be found in Appendix F. Broadly speaking, they are based on a largely successful record search for every hospitalization reported during the two years plus some records found by special search (for example, of those who died) and augmented by a "correction factor"

67. Citywide comparison of study (A and B) and control (C) groups: admissions to general hospitals, by group and year (rates per 1,000).

Group	Admissions	Days	Average stay
First year			
A (appointment)	201	2,610	13.0
B (demand)	210	2,838	13.5
C (control)	170	2,467	14.5
Second year			
A (appointment)	149	1,799	12.1
B (demand)	151	2,532	16.8
C (control)	102	1,510	14.8
National Health Survey, 1962	132.3	905	7.6

that adds in a proportion of the admissions reported but for which no record was found. The amount added in by the "correction factor" is shown in Appendix Tables A-34 and A-36.

From Table 67 it appears that, with one exception, all groups in both years had an above-average use of in-hospital services. The one exception is the C group in the second year; they had fewer admissions than the national average but, on the other hand, their average length of stay was so long that they did receive more bed-days of care than a national cross-section of people in the same year.

To see more clearly the differences between the A, B, and C groups, it seems desirable to separate out the admissions for childbirth, because they constitute a sizable number of the admissions, but their incidence would not be particularly influenced by the medical care system available to the patients (unless a program of birth control, which is a different issue, were offered). Appendix Table A-35 shows that there are indeed no consistent differences in number of deliveries or length of stay for childbirth in the A, B, and C groups.

Analysis will henceforth be concentrated on the admissions to general hospitals for reasons other than childbirth, in an effort to investigate and explain the differences between the three groups (Table 68). It is hard to know how to interpret these differences. It could be that under the existing system (control group C), the patient is least likely to be hospitalized at an early stage of disease; hence in the first year there are the smallest number of hospitalizations but the longest average length of stay. In the second year, when many patients would be off welfare and the special elements of welfare medical care (panel physician home

68. Admissions to general hospitals citywide, by group and year, deliveries excluded (rates per 1,000).

Group	Admissions	Days	Average stay
First year			
A (appointment)	160	2,386	14.9
B (demand)	172	2,646	15.3
C (control)	130	2,249	17.4
Second year			
A (appointment)	124	1,665	13.4
B (demand)	131	2,388	18.2
C (control)	80	1,418	17.6

visits; reimbursed, and hence free, clinic visits at voluntary hospitals; and so on) are no longer available in the control group, very few people are hospitalized, and those that are stay slightly longer than those admitted in the first year. Thus it seems that, aside from the stimulus of a welfare application, with its disability evaluations and referrals for pressing health problems and additional services made available only to those on relief, the indigent seem to reach the hospital in-service only when very sick; hence the low admission rate but long stays in the C group during the second year.

In the A group, on the other hand, hospitalization in both years seems to be more accessible; more people are hospitalized for a shorter average length of stay than in the control group. The number of admissions declines from first to second year, and so does the average stay; one may tentatively suggest that many of the conditions originally needing attention have now been coped with, hence less care is needed. It is possible, on the other hand, that the type of illness in the A group resulted in this particular pattern. Even with the appointment approach, admission rates and lengths of stay remain far above the national average. There seems no doubt at all, from all the evidence accumulated in this report, that people newly admitted to welfare have greater health needs than the general population. The decline from first to second year in hospital utilization rates for the A group may suggest that early care helps to bring conditions under control more quickly. A third experimental year would have been valuable to see whether this downward trend continued.

The B group is the puzzling group to interpret. Even in the first year they averaged somewhat more admissions and longer stays than the A group, though lower in the latter respect than the control group. In the second year, however, they not only maintained this higher rate of hospitalization, but their length of stay increased so markedly that it exceeded both the A and C groups. A third experimental year might have helped explain this finding. If B group admission rates and length of stay were to decrease in the third year, the conclusion would once again be that the B approach (of leaving it up to patients to initiate care) was less efficient and speedy than the A approach (of starting care with an appointment) in bringing patients the benefits of coordinated care. But third year data is lacking, so one can only speculate on this behavior in the B group.

In a further attempt to understand the behavior of the B group, especially with regard to the increased length of stay in the second year, hospitalizations in general hospitals which lasted 30 days or over were examined separately. Appendix Table A-37 shows that there were indeed more of these long-stay admissions in the B group (especially in the second year) and fewer in the C group. Among the long-term admissions, B group patients did not tend to stay longer than those in the other groups. But the fact that the B group experienced *more* long-term admissions goes a long way to account for the longer average stay for B groups if *all* general admissions are considered together.

Proportion of In-patient Care at the New York Hospital. In Chapter 9 the volume and cost of in-patient care rendered to the study group at the New York Hospital were reviewed in detail. These data must be seen in the wider framework of the study group's total in-patient utilization. Table 69 uses only recorded hospital data: it does not add a correction factor for hospitalizations that may have been missed at hospitals other than the New York Hospital. It therefore gives a minimum estimate of outside hospitalization and a maximum estimate of the proportion of in-patient care given at the New York Hospital. Even so, it is clear that a fair amount of in-patient care was given to members of the study group in hospitals other than the New York Hospital. This outside hospitalization, moreover, was by no means limited to the study group patients who did not come to the Project at all.

The utilization patterns for in-patient care, then, differ from those found in out-patient care. In the latter, as Tables 66 and A-33 have demonstrated, most of the study group care given outside the Project was to study group members who did not come to the Project at all.

69. General hospitalizations citywide (deliveries excluded) in the A and B study groups, showing the proportion provided by the New York Hospital (in per cent).

Hospital	First year		Second year	
	A	B	A	B
Admissions at:				
New York Hospital	59	50	53	39
Other hospitals: patients who came	16	18	23	19
Other hospitals: patients who didn't come	25	32	24	42
Total	100	100	100	100
Days at:				
New York Hospital	46	41	43	39
Other hospitals: patients who came	33	22	34	28
Other hospitals: patients who didn't come	21	37	23	33
Total	100	100	100	100

Where those who came to the Project received care elsewhere as well, analysis of the 100-case subsample suggested that it happened either before or after attendance at the New York Hospital, seldom simultaneously.

The in-patients, on the other hand, were often hospitalized both at the New York Hospital and elsewhere during the same period. There were a variety of reasons. It sometimes happened when the patient needed a psychiatric hospitalization (in a general hospital such as Bellevue) or a long general admission exceeding the 60 days the New York Hospital was able to offer. For instance, one elderly lady spent 15 days in the New York Hospital for a cholecystectomy but later spent 5 months in Metropolitan Hospital with metastatic carcinoma of the breast. Another common reason for admissions elsewhere was that the city ambulance followed routine procedure and insisted on taking the patient to its own district hospital, despite his protest that he wanted to go to the New York Hospital. This situation could be documented three times in the 100-case subsample and may have happened on numerous other occasions. One lady in the subsample, who enthusiastically accepted the Project as her main source of care, was admitted to the New York Hospital once but was also admitted to three other hospitals during the two years. Her diabetes was apt to get out of control, and on one occasion when she was incoherent, the police called for the ambulance from Grand Central Hospital and took her there against her will. The next time, because she had moved 20 blocks, it was the Metropolitan ambulance that was called, and she was taken to that hospital while protesting that she belonged to the New York Hospital Project. On the third occasion, she was taken ill while visiting a friend at Kingston, New York, and was admitted to a voluntary hospital there.

It seems administratively more difficult then, to coordinate in-patient than out-patient care, especially from a base that does not constitute the usual source of in-patient care for the particular population to be served. Out-patient care remains largely under the control of the individual patient, so that the important objective is to persuade him to accept the system of care being offered. Deciding on where a person is hospitalized, on the other hand, often involves other people besides the patient himself; in particular, it is important to gain the cooperation of those operating the citywide ambulance service.

Chronic Institutional Care. Chronic institutional care proved to be the kind of medical care most difficult to document accurately. There were three reasons: (1) Chronic institutionalization often made it impossible to interview the respondent. (None were interviewed in state mental hospitals. About one third to one half were approached in chronic hospitals and nursing homes; utilization data were obtained from the staff when the patient was too sick or disoriented to be interviewed.) Many patients who went into chronic institutions during the Project remained there for the rest of the study period. The home interviews were thus less helpful in documenting this kind of care than they were in measuring short-term admissions and doctor visits. (2) It was hard to obtain complete records, especially on state mental hospitalizations and on home care. (3) Some of the respondents who "disappeared" and could not be located for second and third wave interviews may have entered chronic institutions, but their names could not be checked through all the possible institutions.

The tables presented below represent a best estimate of the number of patients who received chronic care during the experimental period, with a very rough estimate of total days. Most admissions to long-term institutions were learned of when Project staff checked with welfare and other possible sources of information for the respondent's latest address, in preparation for the second and third home interviews or from these interviews when NORC found no one at the expected address and traced their whereabouts from relatives and neighbors, or from the death certificates of those who died, or from hospital records. All these sources of information were similar for study and control group patients, so the differences discovered are unlikely to be entirely explained by more complete reporting for the study group. (They could be part of the explanation for nursing home care, because study group patients in or entering nursing homes were automatically referred by the Welfare Department to the Project. But a very careful search from all other sources was undertaken for the control group.)

It seems clear from Table 70 that more persons in the study group than in the control group reached chronic institutions during the two year period. (A few, mainly in nursing homes, were already in the institution at intake.) The difference between A, B, and C groups holds for every kind of institution studied, with B always in an intermediate position between A and C. If the pattern of admissions over the two

70. Citywide comparison of study (A and B) and control (C) groups: persons admitted to long-term institutions in two years (rates per 1,000).

Group	State mental hospital	Chronic hospital	Nursing home	Home care	Any of these institutions
A (appointment)	17	9	15	7	45[a]
B (demand)	15	8	12	5	38
C (control)	10	7	9	4	26

[a]Totals do not necessarily add across, because a few patients were in more than one kind of institution.

year period (Appendix Table A-38) is taken into account, there do not seem to be any consistent differences in timing between the three groups, merely *more* of all kinds of chronic hospitalization in the study group, especially in A.

The difference in chronic care days between study and control group (Table 71) seems to be as large as the difference in persons admitted. Unlike the acute hospitalizations, however, where B consistently experienced more bed-days than A, the reverse seems to be true here. Group A totals slightly more days than B each year, but C is very much lower than either. As might be expected, there is more chronic hospitalization in the second year than the first; but the rise is roughly proportional in all three groups.

71. Days in long-term institutions, by group and year (rates per 1,000).

Group	State mental hospital	Chronic hospital	Nursing home	Home care	Any of these institutions
First year					
A (appointment)	1,953	338	1,998	1,299	5,588
B (demand)	1,546	978	2,350	493	5,369
C (control)	1,256	88	1,732	760	3,836
Second year					
A (appointment)	2,918	953	3,272	1,103	8,246
B (demand)	3,123	1,300	3,098	381	7,902
C (control)	1,761	740	1,797	409	4,707

In Chapter 9 careful cost analysis of the New York Hospital by
Arthur Andersen & Co. provided an accurate determination of the cost
of each medical service available there to Project patients. This chapter
is based on cost data provided from a variety of sources and is of
varying degrees of precision. The comparison of study and control
groups in terms of estimated costs is of such importance that considerable effort was warranted in obtaining the best possible bases for costs
of services rendered under the two systems. The final sums, however,
should be judged as estimated trends rather than as absolute comparisons.

Services and supplies are the input of the medical care system. A
comparison of the two systems of care can be made with this input
expressed in monetary terms. There are several reasons for trying to
provide the best possible estimate of the cost of coordinated medical
care: (1) The share of total community expenditures devoted to health
care and the allocation among various medical services require documentation for intelligent choice between alternative systems of care. (2)
When a contract for comprehensive services to a defined population is
to be made, accurate information concerning the cost of the services to
be provided is essential. Purchase of medical care through insurance
prepayment has increased public concern in the price of these services.
(3) Objective evaluation of the feasibility of new systems of organizing
medical care (the Project study group, for example) requires comparison of cost and outcome (availability and effectiveness of care) with
that of the existing system (control group).

Comparison of *total* study group cost with *total* control group cost
was a major goal of the research. It requires an accurate determination
of the utilization of *all* medical services during the two years under
study. The multitude of services and institutions serving both groups
has been detailed; the methods used to obtain accurate information
about utilization have been described. The problem is how to obtain
reasonable cost figures for the many different services provided by
many different institutions. The difficulties of obtaining detailed cost
accounting for even a limited group of services within one institution
were great (see Chapter 9). Limitations of method and resources would
clearly make it impossible to carry this process through for the great
range of services provided by many institutions to the 2,504 individuals
in the study group and the 1,685 individuals in the control group. A
method was needed for making a useful comparison of the cost of
services to each group using available cost information. Despite recognized limitations in the available data, the aim was to obtain estimated
cost data that would be generally comparable.

The main source of cost data was that provided by the United Hospital Fund for voluntary hospitals. Some of the other sources included the Department of Hospitals for municipal hospitals; the Department of Health for non-hospital clinics; the Department of Welfare for eye and dental clinics; the State Department of Mental Hygiene for mental hospitals and aftercare clinics. Details of the sources of unit cost data may be found in Appendix E.

The United Hospital Fund made available the unit costs for voluntary hospitals, both in-patient day and out-patient visit. UHF calculates the average cost for each member hospital on the basis of detailed information supplied annually by the hospital through a 40-page questionnaire that constitutes a comprehensive report of its total income and expenditures. Costs for the calendar year 1962 were used.

It should be borne in mind throughout this chapter that the need for comparability between study and control group necessitated using these less precise estimates of cost with medical care utilization data as reported by the welfare case respondent rather than data recorded in a hospital chart -- even for the New York Hospital, where precise information was available. For this reason, cost of New York Hospital care per person at risk as estimated in this chapter, where it is set in the context of *total* cost of care per study group person at risk, is not exactly the same as the very precise estimate arrived at in Chapter 9.

Unit costs for municipal and state institutions were obtained from the responsible department (for details see Appendix E). Because actual daily cost data for nursing home care is not available, reimbursement to these private institutions by the Department of Welfare has been used as the basis for this portion of the computation. The same method was used for care provided by welfare panel physicians.

Out-patient Services

Ambulatory services have been grouped into three categories for analysis:

Hospital Clinics. This category includes out-patient department and emergency room care at city and voluntary hospitals.

Non-hospital Clinics. Department of Health clinics (child health, chest, dental, and others), Department of Welfare dental clinics and eye clinics, aftercare psychiatric clinics, and all other non-hospital clinics are grouped in this category.

Non-clinic Care. Included are home and office visits from private physicians (privately arranged and with the cost actually borne by the patient), services of welfare panel physicians (in general available only to control group patients because the Project was designed to take over this function) and home visits by New York Hospital project physicians.

The 1962 unit cost per visit used (see Appendix E) was as follows:

Hospital clinics

New York Hospital clinic (including emergency room)	$10.78
Mount Sinai clinic (including emergency room)	10.78
Other voluntary hospitals combined (including emergency room)	9.46
Bellevue Hospital clinic	6.59
Metropolitan Hospital clinic	6.59
Other city hospitals combined	6.94
City hospital emergency room	8.27

Non-hospital clinics

Department of Health child health	3.74
Department of Health chest	9.89
Department of Health dental	7.83
Department of Health other	7.00
Department of Welfare eye	7.52
Department of Welfare dental	7.85
Aftercare (per patient per year)	200.00
Other dental clinics	7.00
Other non-hospital clinics	7.00

Non-clinic care

Private physician—home	10.00
Private physician—office	5.00
Welfare panel physician	4.00
Project physician home visit	4.00

The cost for a particular clinic service was obtained by multiplying utilization, measured as described in Chapter 10, by the above unit cost (detailed breakdown is given in Appendix E). To provide comparability between groups of somewhat uneven size, cost was calculated per individual at risk. Naturally, one would expect from the utilization data that study group costs would be greater. Table 72 gives the estimated costs for the study and control groups.

It is clear that cost of ambulant care for the A group was over 50 per cent greater than for the control group during the first year and almost twice as great (93 per cent higher) during the second year. During both years the B group cost was intermediate: 23 per cent greater than the control group for the first year and 33 per cent greater for the second year.

If the cost of hospital clinic utilization is separated from the cost of total ambulatory care, the cost of care rendered the study group is found to exceed that secured by the control group by a greater

72. Citywide comparison of study (A and B) and control (C) groups: calculated cost of ambulant care per person at risk, by group and year (in dollars).

Source of treatment	Study group		Control group (C)
	A	B	
First year			
Hospital clinics	66	51	36
Non-hospital clinics	7	7	9
Non-clinic care	2	1	3
Total	75	59	48
Second year			
Hospital clinics	54	37	25
Non-hospital clinics	3	2	2
Non-clinic care	1	1	3
Total	58	40	30

magnitude than the percentages reported above for *total* ambulatory care. The cost of care given the A group exceeded that for the C group by 83 per cent and 116 per cent in the first and second year respectively, and the cost of care for the B group exceeded C group cost by 41 per cent and 48 per cent in the consecutive years. Of all the sources of ambulant care enumerated in Table 72, it is apparent that hospital clinic care contributes most to the disparity in cost of care between the study and control groups. The greater cost of care for this source is attributable to the impact of the invitation for complete care extended by the Project. The difference in cost in A group as compared with B group relates to the effects of the two different methods of invitation employed.

For both the study groups, hospital clinic costs represented over 85 per cent of ambulatory care during the first year and over 93 per cent during the second year. For the control group, non-hospital clinics and private (including panel) physicians contributed a greater share of cost than they did for study patients.

During the first year the New York Hospital accounted for 62 per cent of the cost of ambulatory care for the A group, but only 43 per cent for the B group (Appendix Table A-39). Voluntary hospitals together accounted for less than a third of the ambulatory care cost for the control group who received the largest single portion of their care from city hospital clinics.

During the second year the cost of ambulatory services decreased, and the New York Hospital provided a greater proportion of the study group's ambulatory care than during the first year, that is, 13 per cent more for the A group and 8 per cent more for the B group.

In-patient Services

In-patient services have been grouped into two broad categories.

General Hospitals. Voluntary and city hospitals are analyzed separately and the hospitals giving the greatest share of care are considered individually. The 1962 United Hospital Fund calculated cost per hospital day was employed for voluntary hospitals, and unit costs for municipal hospitals were supplied by the Department of Hospitals (see Appendix E).

New York Hospital	$46.44
Mount Sinai Hospital	45.29
Other voluntary hospitals (average)	37.26
Bellevue Hospital	41.35
Metropolitan Hospital	38.59
Other city hospitals (average)	38.88

Chronic Care Institutions. Three categories were used and cost figures were derived as detailed in Appendix E.

State mental hospitals	$ 6.39
Nursing homes	8.71
Chronic care hospitals	21.87

Table 73 shows the largest single cost unit in the medical care package: general hospital in-patient care. Average estimated per person cost for study group A was $111, for study group B $120, and $100 for the control group during the first year. During the second year the disparity was considerably greater with A group and C group costs dropping 30 per cent and 40 per cent respectively but B group costs falling only 12 per cent. Thus, during both years, but to a much more pronounced extent during the second year, general hospital care for the demand group (B) was greater than for the appointment group (A). This is in marked contrast to out-patient average cost as previously presented.

Estimated costs for chronic care were markedly higher during the second year (Table 74). (As indicated in Chapter 10, accurate utilization data on chronic hospitalization has been extremely difficult to obtain and these data are less accurate than the previous material.)

The increase seems particularly marked in the appointment group (A), whose costs almost doubled (from $38 to $75). Costs for A group and B group in the second year are equal ($75), but the B group began from a much higher first year base of $53. This high cost in the demand

73. Calculated cost of general hospital in-patient care citywide per person at risk, by group and year (in dollars).

Hospital	Study group		Control group (C)
	A	B	
First year			
New York Hospital	48	44	4
Mount Sinai	3	8	17
Other voluntary	12	14	15
Bellevue	33	35	34
Metropolitan	14	18	28
Other city	1	1	2
Total	111	120	100
Second year			
New York Hospital	31	35	3
Mount Sinai	1	5	4
Other voluntary	9	22	14
Bellevue	27	24	18
Metropolitan	6	15	18
Other city	3	4	3
Total	77	105	60

group (B) in the first year was contributed primarily by more chronic hospital admissions. Costs for C group, consistently lower than A or B, increased by over 50 per cent in the second year. A gradual increase in institutional care seems inevitable in a group as sick as this Project population has proved to be. A possible interpretation of Table 74 is that the Project patients in the study group (A and B) were moved more quickly into appropriate levels of care than were patients in the control group.

Additional Medical Care Cost

A comparison between medical administrative costs for the control group and the study group presents major difficulties. A limited amount of medical care coordination for the control group was undertaken within the Welfare Department. Because this coordination falls among other Welfare Department responsibilities, an exact cost determination is difficult to obtain. An estimated cost for this of $7.70 per

74. Calculated cost of chronic institutional care citywide per person at risk, by group and year (in dollars).

Hospital	Study group		Control group (C)
	A	B	
First year			
State mental hospitals	14	11	7
Nursing homes	17	21	15
Chronic hospitals	7	21	7
Total	38	53	29
Second year			
State mental hospitals	19	20	12
Nursing homes	29	27	16
Chronic hospitals	27	28	17
Total	75	75	45

year for each individual in the control group was obtained.[1] A much more ambitious program of medical care administration and coordination was undertaken for the study group and the cost is detailed in Chapter 9 (see Table 59). Project staff costs were determined as an average annual cost of $26 for each individual at risk in the study group. This cost, however, included actual medical care as well as coordination and administration.

The cost of in-patient and out-patient care contains expenditure for administrative services. No attempt has been made to separate this expenditure from other costs. However, the task of coordinating individual and family care and providing continuity of information and follow-up through a team of nurses, social workers, clerical, and administrative personnel, as well as physicians, is essential in an increasingly complex medical world. Though the precise cost of coordination could not be separated, its importance demands an effort to include it in the cost analysis. The integrative system that was developed probably accounts for about 10 per cent of the total cost of all medical care for the study group.

1. Arthur Andersen & Co. studied the medical unit at the Yorkville Welfare Center from January to June 1962: $15.24 was found to be the administrative unit cost per case. Mr. Henry Rosner, assistant to the commissioner, Department of Welfare, supplied the number of welfare recipients administered by the Yorkville Center, for the same period. The average for the six month period is 12,824 people in 6,488 cases. There were 1.98 individuals per case. A unit cost of $7.70 per person was derived for welfare medical administration.

Total Estimated Cost of Care

The average total estimated cost of medical care per person at risk is summarized in Table 75. During the first year the cost of care for both study groups was higher than for the control group: A group costs per person at risk were 35 per cent higher than C, B group costs were 39 per cent higher. During the second year this discrepancy between study and control group costs increased; the difference rose to 64 per cent and 69 per cent above control group costs for A and B respectively. The higher cost in the study group holds for every single kind of medical care cost.

One fact that stands out from Table 75, however, is that the A group approach of beginning care by sending the patient an appointment proved no more expensive, once the whole spectrum of services is reviewed, than the B group method of leaving the patient to come in on demand. Even in the first year, A group total costs were slightly lower than B; and this situation persists into the second year. If chronic institutional care is omitted, then A group costs declined considerably more from first to second year than did B group costs.

Moreover, some interesting differences in the distribution of A and B group costs were noted. The costs of ambulatory care were greater in the A group than the B group, and the costs of in-patient care were

75. Calculated cost of total medical care citywide per person at risk, by group and year (in dollars).

Type of care	Study group		Control group (C)
	A	B	
First year			
Ambulant care	75	60	48
General in-patient care	111	120	100
Chronic institutional care	38	53	29
Coordination administration	26	26	8
Total	250	259	185
Second year			
Ambulant care	58	40	30
General in-patient care	77	105	60
Chronic institutional care	75	75	45
Coordination administration	26	26	8
Total	236	246	143

greater in B than A. This trend grew in the second year, suggesting the possibility that a more complete and early use of out-patient facilities may reduce in-patient costs.

Discussion

We have attempted to calculate the cost of the medical care process and to compare the study and control group in this respect. This comparison must be accompanied by a comparison of the outcome of the process. In subsequent chapters an attempt will be made to assess results both subjectively, as reflected in the satisfaction of those who received and those who gave medical care, and objectively, insofar as it is reflected in tangible results. In short, how much more does this system of medical care cost than the existing system and how much more is the community getting in return? It appears that this question, and many others related to it, can only be answered in relative terms, that is, by comparing one method or system with another. Because detailed cost accounting information for each institution did not exist, the Project was forced to construct a method of obtaining calculated costs that would allow estimated comparisons.

Limiting the study period to two years imposed certain restrictions. When accepted on the welfare rolls, many individuals had a backlog of untended medical problems; in fact, some were forced to apply for welfare for health reasons. Thus, extensive and costly services were required on enrollment. One would hope that at least in certain age categories, improved care would gradually be reflected in a reduced requirement for the more expensive in-patient services. However, the short period of time covered by the study as well as present technical limitations in dealing adequately with serious psychiatric, degenerative, and neoplastic diseases did not make it possible to demonstrate this effect. The data suggest that coordinated care may tend to move patients through the medical care system to the level of care appropriate for them more quickly then uncoordinated care.

Unit cost per service is considerably higher in the university teaching hospital. Because the Project was based at such an institution and the control group received a greater proportion of its care at municipal hospitals, the study group was at some disadvantage with regard to an estimated cost comparison.

It is a measure of the complexity and diversity of medical care services rendered in a large city that even those members of the study group who regarded the New York Hospital Project as their primary source of medical care received many services elsewhere. The reasons have been discussed previously. It is of interest that of the $250 calculated average cost for group A during the first year less than half was incurred at the New York Hospital ($48 was contributed by the New York Hospital in-patient utilization, $46 for New York Hospital out-patient visits, and $26 for Project administration). These conditions demonstrate the need to study the entire range of services obtained by patients in order to assess the dimensions of cost.

Welfare medical care for 500,000 individuals in New York City is currently rendered by the Department of Welfare (through vendor payment), Department of Health, Department of Hospitals, State Department of Mental Hygiene, as well as some philanthropic and private sources. Because these organizations also take care of many others, the portion of their budget to be attributed to the 500,000 welfare recipients is difficult to determine.

The study confirms that medical care is expensive, that costs are rising at a rapid rate, and that attempts to improve medical care increase costs. To what extent these costs are necessary or desirable is beyond the scope of this discussion, but in a period of rapidly rising expectations on the part of those who receive medical care and those who render it, rising cost appears to be inevitable.

Because of a rapidly rising economic spiral and many competing demands, methods are required for comparing and assessing the cost and effectiveness of present and future systems of rendering care. What is the potential of preventive services? To what extent can less expensive services, such as a home care program, relieve the pressure on more costly services, such as in-patient care in the general hospital? What role can electronic data storing and processing play? Which organizational pattern allows the optimal use of highly trained personnel? In this time of rapid change many such questions press for carefully documented answers.

Health services are aimed at the prevention, control, or cure of disease and at rehabilitation of the patient. The performance of the service, however, is not synonymous with the accomplishment of its purpose. Evaluation of health services, commonly described as determination of the quality of medical care, often stops short at assessing the performance of the service itself. Yet the ultimate criterion is the effectiveness of the service in achieving the goal toward which it is aimed.

Measuring effectiveness of medical care in terms of goals or end results presents enormous problems. First, health services include an almost infinite number of different processes – for example, cardiac surgery, psychotherapy, the immunization of children, the control of air pollution, the treatment of diabetes; and each process requires a different measuring tool. General rules may be helpful but are unreliable for precise measurement. It is essential to have both adequate facilities and a sufficient number of appropriately trained personnel, but these alone do not guarantee the effectiveness of the services they provide. Again, highly effective service in one area does not always insure equally effective care in other areas of the same institution; in-patient and out-patient departments in some hospitals differ considerably in the quality of care they provide.

A second and even more complicated characteristic of the health services is their rapid rate of change. The criteria of good care are constantly changing with every new scientific advance. Not only are new preventive, diagnostic, and therapeutic measures continually being discovered, but new illnesses are created by drugs or by air, food, and water pollution -- not to mention the hazards of nuclear fallout. There are whole new areas of preventive medicine made possible by advances in geriatrics, social psychiatry, and mental health. In the treatment of acute illness, evaluation of new procedures is simplified by the shorter time required to judge results. But in the area of chronic disease, which constitutes the major problem today, it is more difficult to judge the extent to which new treatments influence the natural history of the illness. Moreover, some new procedures whose effectiveness has been proven are in short supply and prohibitively expensive: an example would be extra-corporeal dialysis machines for the treatment of glomerulonephritis. Evaluation of the effectiveness of medical care must take into account the extent to which social and moral judgments are involved in determining the availability and distribution of scarce resources.

Finally, one must allow for the fact there is frequently a difference of opinion between the providers and the recipients of health services about the definition of illness and the appropriateness and adequacy of treatment. For instance, patients with emotional problems may consider themselves organically ill, and their opinions about the treatment they should receive and the results that can be achieved may differ markedly from those of the therapist. Another very sensitive area of potential conflict concerns terminally ill patients who, because of recent scientific developments, can sometimes be maintained in a state of biological persistence after the loss of personality. The question of who decides on the desirability of this therapy raises profound moral issues. It also raises questions concerning the appropriateness of using mortality data as indices of quality of care. It has usually been assumed that preventing death or prolonging life is, without qualification, desirable; and few would dispute this if the patient is restored to health and function. Preservation of the life of a severely deformed baby, or prolongation of the life of an adult in a vegetable state of existence, however, may not necessarily deserve to be put on the credit side of the ledger in an examination of the outcome of various systems of health care.

Aware of these conceptual and practical difficulties in assessing quality or effectiveness of medical care, Project staff nevertheless felt the obligation to try to compare the whole study group and control group populations and to look for differences in the medical services they had received and the effect of these services on health, function, or longevity. Three comparative studies were attempted: perinatal care; mortality; persons reporting urinary symptoms on intake on Welfare (see Chapter 13). These studies represent three different approaches. The perinatal studies were concentrated mainly on the provision of health services. The amount, type, and timing of prenatal and post-natal care received by the mothers under the two systems were compared. Outcome, or effect of these services, was only incidentally reviewed in terms of comparing maternal or infant deaths, or infant abnormalities, in study and control group. With the small numbers involved, it was not expected that any significant differences would be found here, although there might well be differences in the kind of care provided.

The mortality study was entirely a study of outcome, that is, death, in the two groups. Discussion will show the difficulty of relating the death to the medical care system in which the patient had previously been situated.

Perinatal Care

There was a total of 163 births in study and control group reported on the home interview at the end of the first year of medical care. One hundred thirty-seven of these births were reported to have taken place in the four most frequently used hospitals: Bellevue, Metropolitan, the

New York Hospital, and Mount Sinai. One birth occurred in Puerto Rico and the remaining births were spread over 12 different hospitals in New York City.

In attempting to verify the reported births, a record search was undertaken at the four major hospitals. Some record, complete or partial, was found for 120 of the deliveries. Appendix Table A-40 shows the extent of success of the record search; it was mainly at Bellevue that difficulty was encountered in locating the charts.

Table 76 shows a comparison of the number of recorded births in the study and control groups at the four major hospitals. The 27 women in the study group who came to the New York Hospital to have their babies delivered represent a real change in the pattern of medical care of the welfare population: only two women in the control group came to the New York Hospital for delivery. On the other hand, the number is small in comparison to the entire study group, because it represents less than a third of the study group deliveries. This proportion reflects the lower response of the families than of the single cases to the invitation to the New York Hospital.

Comparisons were made of obstetrical characteristics of study and control group mothers. These included age of the mother, number of previous births, past history of abortion or premature birth. There were no significant differences between the two groups.

Comparisons were next attempted on the outcome of pregnancy. However, there were too few premature or sick infants to make meaningful comparisons between study and control groups. Specific complications of pregnancy also could not readily be compared because hospital records varied in their descriptions of this, nor did such complications seem to correlate with the outcome of the pregnancy in the small number of cases in which they occurred.

Another area of comparison was utilization patterns in both groups. The average number of antenatal visits in both study and control groups

76. Study and control group births for which records were found, four main hospitals, first year.

Hospital	Study group	Control group	Total
Bellevue	26	22	48
New York Hospital	27	2	29
Metropolitan	18	13	31
Mount Sinai	7	5	12
Total	79	43	120

77. Comparison of selected items of perinatal care in study and control groups, four main hospitals, first year.

Item	Study groups			Control group
	NYH	Other hospitals	Total	
Births with some record	27	51	78	42
Average number of antenatal visits	5.0	7.0	6.2	6.3
Seen first or second trimester	15/26	24/37	39/63	17/29
Post-partum exam 4–8 weeks	15/26	20/43	35/69	13/36
Any visit at same hospital within year	23/26	26/43	49/69	23/36
Baby at same hospital within year	25/27	23/46	48/73	17/35

was very similar (Table 77). Nor was there any significant difference between these groups in the number of patients who came during the first or second trimester of pregnancy. In the study group, 39 out of 63 came for antenatal visits at this stage, compared with 17 out of 29 in the control group.

Patients delivered at the New York Hospital were somewhat more likely to return for post-partum examination four to eight weeks after delivery (15 out of 26 at the New York Hospital, compared with 20 out of 43 in the study group delivered at other hospitals, and 13 out of 36 in the control group). In comparing total visits to the same hospital in the year following delivery, whether for post-partum examination or not, the differences are clearer. Twenty-three out of 26 returned to the New York Hospital in the year following delivery, compared with 26 out of 43 in the study group elsewhere, and 23 out of 36 in the control group. These differences in the New York Hospital patients were not large enough to yield a significant difference between the study group as a whole and the control group.

The last aspect compared (and here the data are very incomplete) was the number of instances in which the infant pediatric care during the first year of life took place at the hospital where the baby was born. Obviously, the alternative to this is not that the infants did not receive care. However, because all these hospitals did have well-baby clinics as well as facilities for sick children, it seemed worthwhile to know whether the children were brought back to the hospitals where they were born. In those of the study group delivered at the New York Hospital, 25 out of 27 were brought back for further care, compared with 23 out of 46 in the study group delivered elsewhere, and 17 out of 35 in the control group. Again, those delivered at the New York Hospital behaved quite differently, but their number was not large enough to cause a difference between the whole study group and the control group.

In conclusion, this limited review of perinatal care suggests that mothers delivered at the New York Hospital showed no demonstrable difference from those delivered elsewhere as regards prenatal care, obstetrical experience, or outcome of pregnancy but that they were more likely than the others to return for post-partum examination and for other health care in the same hospital. They were also far more likely to bring their babies for well-child care at the hospital at which they were delivered. However, only a third of all deliveries in the first year took place at the New York Hospital, a fact that reflects the far greater difficulty in reaching young families living at the extremes of the Yorkville district than in attracting the older, sicker patients living near the hospital. The importance of the Project to perinatal care was therefore limited and there were not significant differences between the *total* study group and the control group, even in the area of post-partum care. Therefore, the study was not extended beyond the four major hospitals or to the births occurring in the second year.

Mortality as a Measure of the Quality of Medical Care

Mortality rates have traditionally been used as one way of assessing the health of a population; measures of this kind are attractive for their simplicity and universality. In seeking ways of measuring the quality of medical care in the Project, it was therefore felt that one measure might be found in the number of deaths of the different sub-groups of this population. In practice, this turned out not to be the case and no differences in mortality were found between study and control groups that could properly be attributed to the effect of the medical care provided. However, analysis of these data appears to demonstrate several of the factors underlying this type of approach and it is essentially from this standpoint that the data are presented. They are of further interest in providing limited mortality statistics for a welfare-supported population.

Reflection on the findings points up the drawbacks of the mortality comparison. First, the population is small and death is a fairly rare event; to what extent will a non-specific death rate really reflect the quality -- or nature -- of the care that was given? How "preventable" were the deaths that occurred? The population was a selected one in the sense that the people were included by virtue of their eligibility for welfare support; they were observed for only a short period of time. Both these factors subsume other factors that could be of greater significance in determining mortality than medical care. In treating overall medical care as an epidemiological variable without further qualifications and in terms of the morbidity of a population like that of New York City it must be recognized that its influence on mortality is likely to be weak in comparison with other factors.

A second difficulty is the lack of comparable data. Death rates for the indigent population are not readily computed, so that it has not been possible to assess these data in terms of comparable groups. The comparisons made here between the Project population and that of New York City are arbitrary. One must again bear in mind that the mortality experienced by the people making up the Project is dependent on the selection criteria of welfare eligibility to an unknown extent and that these legal criteria vary between categories; it is impossible to define the population in terms of its natural characteristics -- which may, in any case, be very diffuse. It is therefore not possible to relate the mortality of the Project population to that of a demographically defined "pool," nor to estimate the "expected" mortality rates.

As far as could be determined, there were 112 deaths in the Project population; these provide a crude annual death rate of 13.4 per 1,000 (Table 78). There are slight, and insignificant, differences between study and control groups, and all the rates are a little higher than the 1963 rate for New York City of 11.4 per 1,000. The closeness of these Project figures to the city rate is coincidental and is dependent on the fact that the age structure of the Project population differs from that of the city: if the age-specific rates shown in Table 79 are examined the impression is very different. At all age groups except the youngest (under 30), there are marked differences between the Project rate and the city rate. The greatest deviation is in the age range 30-69, where the Project exceeds the city rate by a multiple of 2.5; but even in the oldest group (70 or over), the Project rate is considerably higher.

The influence of welfare eligibility becomes evident in Table 80, which expresses mortality in terms of the various welfare categories.

78. Crude mortality rates of Project population, by group, compared with New York City (per 1,000 population per annum).

Group	Rate
A	14.6
B	13.7
C	12.2
All groups	13.4
New York City, 1963	11.4

79. Mortality rates at different ages, Project population compared with New York City.

Age	Rate for Project	Rate for New York City[a]
Less than 30	1.6	2.0
30–49	10.6	4.0
50–69	51.7	18.5
70 or over	105.5	83.6
All ages	13.4	11.4

[a]Based on deaths in 1963 and census data from 1960.

80. Mortality rates of Project population by welfare category.

Category	Rate
Aid to Dependent Children	0.24
Home Relief	7.9
Aid to Disabled, or Blind	60.5
Old Age Assistance, Medical Aid to the Aged	86.8

Aid to Dependent Children, as one might expect, shows a low rate, as does the Home Relief category. In contrast, the various categories supporting the disabled (Aid to the Disabled, Pending Aid to the Disabled, Aid to the Blind) have a very high rate at 60.5 per 1,000. Persons on Old Age Assistance and Medical Aid to the Aged also have a high rate, although when one remembers that recipients in these groups must be aged 65, the rate of 86.8 per 1,000 is not grossly at variance with the city rate of 83.6 for persons aged 70 or over.

Recalling our earlier questioning of the applicability of mortality as an indicator throughout the population, it is interesting that almost 80 per cent of the deaths occurred among persons supported by the various Aid to Disabled and Old Age Assistance categories. These groups comprised only 14 per cent of the overall Project population.

The principal causes of death are summarized in Table 81. These are much as one might imagine them to be and their frequency is similar to that for the older population of the city in general. The numbers in each grouping are small for statistical purposes, but it is notable that 5 of the 11 deaths from respiratory disease were certified as due to

81. Causes of death in Project population (study and control groups combined).

Cause of death	Number	Per cent
Cardiovascular diseases	29	25.9
Neoplasms	23	20.5
Vascular lesions of the CNS	10	8.9
Respiratory diseases[a,b]	11	9.8
Accidents/suicide	9	8.0
Gastro-intestinal diseases[b]	7	6.3
Other diseases	9	8.0
Cause not determined	14	12.5
Total	112	100.0

[a]Includes five deaths from pulmonary tuberculosis.

[b]Exclusive of neoplasms.

pulmonary tuberculosis. (The age - adjusted rate for New York City for 1959–1961 was 7.3 per 100,000.) A possible interpretation of this high frequency is that welfare support is a socioeconomic correlate of advanced tuberculosis and that this observation is an example of the way in which welfare eligibility and illness are interrelated.

The place in which the individual died is perhaps some indicator of the type of care he received before death; for a variety of technical reasons it was not possible to obtain record abstracts of the care administered during the terminal illness, but Table 82 contrasts the place of death of the two main Project groups with estimates for New York City in 1963. About half the deaths in both the study and control groups of the Project occurred in either city or state hospitals -- an excess of about 20 per cent over the city proportion, where a greater percentage of deaths occurring in voluntary institutions is found. A quarter of the deaths in each group happened in the patients' homes.

A curious difference between the study and control group concerns deaths in voluntary hospitals. Roughly the same proportion of deaths occurred in these institutions in each group (and this is also true for city hospitals), but two thirds of the study group deaths in voluntary hospitals occurred at the New York Hospital, compared with none of the control group deaths. Thus, the pattern of deaths in city hospitals seems not to have been affected by the Project, but a "shift" appears to have occurred from other voluntary hospitals to the New York Hospital of study group patients who subsequently died. Although the available

82. Place of death, Project population compared with New York City (in per cent).

Place of death	Study group (N=71)	Control group (N=41)	New York City, 1963 (N=88,026)
City and state hospitals	48	51	30
Voluntary hospitals (not NYH)	6	15	31
New York Hospital	11	0	
Nursing home	6	5	11
At home	25	27	26
Other places	4	2	2
Total, N=100 per cent	100	100	100

facts cannot support such a speculation, it does provide an example of the possible uses of mortality data in observing patterns of utilization. It would be interesting to explore in more detail the characteristics of the people dying in different places and the factors that determine where they die.

Other uses for mortality data are cases with or without autopsy and cases referred to the medical examiner. Just over one fifth (23 per cent) of the persons dying on the Project had post-mortem examinations and rather less than one third of the cases were referred to the medical examiner. Both these proportions are comparable to those for the city. The proportion of Project deaths that occurred at home and were also referred to the medical examiner, however, was markedly higher than the comparable figures for the city (73 per cent in contrast to 48 per cent for the city). Twenty-eight per cent of the deaths were referred to the medical examiner (the general rate for New York City is about 30 per cent). Seventy-three per cent--23 out of 29--of deaths occurring in the home were referred to the medical examiner (the New York City rate is 48 per cent). The certified causes of death in these cases were: cardiovascular disease--10 cases; cirrhosis of the liver--2 cases; other diseases--4 cases. Again, lack of data relating to the terminal illness is a handicap and no explanation for this excess can be found; but the certified causes of death in some of these cases do seem to raise questions about prior medical care. Why, for example, should deaths certified as being due to pulmonary tuberculosis or cirrhosis of the liver be referred to the medical examiner? Mortality data on their own cannot enlarge on these questions, but this is another example of their utility in suggesting areas for closer investigation.

Discussions of the welfare population sometimes create the impression that people may come on to welfare toward the end of a long chronic illness and that welfare support may be a prelude to death. The death rates and causes of death shown earlier in the tables might tend to support this view, but Table 83 demonstrates that this was not the case if the overall population over the two year duration of the Project is considered. The number of deaths in each of the six months of the Project period is roughly the same. On the other hand, something of this effect is seen when the deaths are further divided by age (Table 84). There is a significantly greater number of "early" deaths in the

83. Distribution of deaths during the period of the Project.

Months on Project before death	Number	Per cent
Less than 6	26	23
6–11	25	22
12–17	32	29
18 or more	26	23
Not known	3	3
Total	112	100

84. Age in relation to length of time on the Project before death.[a]

	Time on Project					
	Less than one year		One year or more		Total	
Age	Number	Per cent	Number	Per cent	Number	Per cent
Under 60	24	63	14	37	38	100
60 or over	27	38	44	62	71	100
Total	51	46	58	54	109[b]	100

[a]$\chi^2 = 7.26$, $df = 1$, $p < 0.01$.

[b]Date of three deaths unknown.

younger population (which is, in this context, essentially the Aid to the Disabled group). This is a further illustration of the way in which different selection criteria at different ages influence the applicability of outcome factors like mortality in its relation to the provision of medical care. A proper application can probably be reached only by relating these deaths to a more naturally defined population of which each welfare category forms an unknown part.

The relationship between the utilization of Project services and death is obviously a complex one. One is here dealing with a range of sociological and epidemiological variables that may influence both utilization and death in varying degrees: differences in the duration, severity, and complexity of illness, in the ability or willingness of the individual to utilize medical care, and in the degree to which persons with illnesses likely to be fatal have already established stable patterns of care are examples of the factors that might operate in this relationship. A simple statement of mortality in those who did and did not use the Project is shown in Table 85. This table is restricted to persons supported by the Aid to Disabled and Old Age Assistance categories and shows a significantly smaller proportion of deaths among those who came to the New York Hospital. At first sight, these figures speak well for the aims of the Project. However, there seems to be an alternative explanation: the possibility that chronic disease leading to death and failure to respond to the Project invitation were associated in a proportion of these cases. In using death as an indicator of the effectiveness of care, a more precise estimate of the nature and extent of morbidity is needed at the outset of the study than was possible in the present experiment. Only by having such a "primary" definition can divergent patterns of behavior be contrasted and different groups be standardized with respect to relevant variables.

Attitudes to health and to medical care also influence patterns of utilization, just as the presence or absence of disease will influence attitudes. Table 86 demonstrates that these influences can also be

85. Mortality in those members of the study group who did and did not come to the New York Hospital for care (persons on AD, AB, OAA, and MAA only, in per cent).[a]

Use	Died	Did not die
Came to NYH (N=170)	11.3	88.7
Did not come to NYH (N=47)	20.8	79.2
All study group	14.2	85.8

[a] $x^2 = 6.61, df = 1, p < 0.01$.

86. Selected questions from the first attitude questionnaire comparing responses of those who did and did not die (persons on AD, AB, OAA, and MAA only).

	Percentage distribution	
Respondents' rating of own health	Died (N=92)	Did not die (N=824)
Question		
Excellent	8	9
Good	18	24
Fair	20	37
Poor	53	30
Frequency of thinking about own health		
Fairly often	59	52
Once in a while	17	21
Hardly ever	24	26
Saw doctor in previous year		
Yes	90	73
No	10	27
Satisfaction with the doctor		
Entirely satisfied	84	76
Some things not satisfactory	16	24
Preference for type of medical setting		
Clinic or emergency room	49	36
Private doctor	41	54
Don't know	10	10
Opinion as to whether *most people* in this country would be better off in next two years		
Better off	32	36
About the same	25	24
Worse off	15	20
Don't know	28	19
Opinion as to whether *respondent* will be better off in the next two years		
Better off	27	43
About the same	33	28
Worse off	12	13
Don't know	28	16

observed in mortality statistics by comparing the responses of persons who did or did not die to items selected from the questionnaire administered at the time that the individual entered the Project. Again, the tables are restricted to people in the Aid to the Disabled, Old Age Assistance, and Medical Aid to the Aged welfare categories. Those who died tended to rate their health poorly more often that did those who did not die, but they were no more likely to think about it often. They tended to be more satisfied with their doctor and, as a group, had somewhat different preferences for the type of medical setting in which they received their care; half the respondents who later died said they preferred a clinic or emergency room compared to just over a third of those who did not die -- a greater proportion of whom preferred the services of a private doctor. The people who died also differed from their fellows in their view of *themselves.* Asked whether "most people in this country" would be better or worse off in the next two years, the responses of both groups showed no differences. However, when a similar question was asked about their own expected financial position, only 27 per cent of the death group -- in contrast to 43 per cent of the remainder -- felt that they would be better off.

Medical care, viewed epidemiologically, has the potential to alter the outcome of a situation of itself, but this potential will be dependent to some degree on the interaction of the medical care "variable" with other variables which, in their turn, can also act directly to influence the outcome. If an attempt is to be made to use mortality experience as a measure of the influence of contrasting patterns of medical care, then an estimate of the strength of this interaction and of the strength of medical care as an independent variable in relation to other variables would seem to be prerequisites. The present study demonstrates some aspects of these prerequisites but also points out some of the difficulties in achieving them. The need for a description of the population at the time the sample is drawn raises difficulties in assessing the "degree of severity" of complex clinical situations and then of aggregating patients who may be very different in many senses. It is desirable also to be able to make some form of assessment of population in respect to its temporal progression: in thinking of mortality in a welfare population, what proportion of the initial sample is improving and what proportion is deteriorating? And at what rate? At what stage in the process are we applying medical care? Finally, it seems necessary to have an appreciation of medical care as a part of the sociocultural environment of the population and to be able to judge one's measuring instrument in this broader context.

All these are large questions in themselves. However, the simpler use of tools like the mortality rate (drawing attention to differences between population groups and leading to other methods of investigation) should not be disparaged. The difference in death rates between the Project and the city population in the 30-69 age range would seem to be an example of this function.

13 | Measuring Effectiveness of Medical Care II: Medical Care as a Problem-solving Activity

The available methods of measuring "quality" or effectiveness of medical care have been seen in the preceding chapters to be inadequate for a useful comparison of study group and control group. In order to devise a more satisfactory and comprehensive method, medical care was analyzed as a problem-solving activity. Seven stages in the solution of a medical problem were considered: recognition by the patient of the existence of a problem; availability and use of help; ability of the physician to recognize that a problem exists (identification of the symptoms and signs); categorization of the problem (diagnosis) and possibly identification of precipitating factors (etiology); action on the problem (treatment); resolution of the problem; determination of whether the problem has been solved (follow-up). By starting with a specific symptom or group of symptoms, it is possible to analyze the successive stages of medical care using this conceptual framework. Two comparable populations, differing only in the system by which they receive care, can then be compared (study group and control group).

In the health questionnaire, administered just before intake to those aged 18 or over, two questions concerning urinary tract symptoms were asked, and the positive responses are tabulated in Table 87. These are the individuals who recognized the existence of a problem when asked about it. Their medical experiences during the subsequent two years are the subject of our analysis. As can be seen in Table 88, females outnumbered males in the under 50 age group; the reverse was true over age 50.

The first step in following up the persons who had reported urinary symptoms at intake was to see how many of them saw a doctor in the two year study period. The home interviews at the end of the first and second year, supplemented by a record search at the hospitals each had reported using (in addition to a search in the four most-used hospitals for records for those who could not be interviewed on one or both

87. Adults in study and control group who reported urinary symptoms at intake (N=1,980).

Symptom	Study group	Control group
Trouble with urination only	84	61
Blood in urine only	0	6
Both symptoms	20	9
Total, either or both symptoms	104	76

88. Age and sex distribution of adults reporting urinary symptoms, at intake.

Age at intake	Male	Female
14–19	0	4
20–29	4	23
30–39	12	26
40–49	8	14
50–59	21	14
60–69	10	14
70–79	15	8
80 or over	2	5
Total	72	108

89. Apparent use of medical care in the following two years by persons reporting urinary symptoms at intake, by group.

Use of medical care	Study group Number	Study group Per cent	Control group Number	Control group Per cent
Hospital record of medical care found	86	83	48	63
Reported hospital use, no record found	12	11	13	17
Reported hospital use, record found, no utilization during study	1		2	
Reported no medical care	3	6	3	20
Not interviewed and no record found	2		10	
Total	104	100	76	100

waves), yielded the results summarized in Table 89. Eighty-three per cent of the study group had hospital records showing they had seen a doctor during the two years, compared with only 63 per cent of the control group. This is a statistically significant difference and constitutes the sharpest difference between study and control group in this study. The study and control group systems of care seem to differ most widely in the second stage of the problem-solving activity, namely, in the availability of medical service and the patient's use of it.

Table 90 shows the institutions used by the various people whose records could be found. The majority of the study group did attend the New York Hospital, but very few of the control group did so. A number of patients used more than one hospital during the two years. Altogether, just over half of those using hospitals had been out-patients only.

When the records were searched, the first object of concern was whether or not the examining physician had elicited the urinary symptom. Because diagnosis relies on history and physical examination, we have tabulated the record of this basic information (Table 91). The existence of a urinary complaint was recorded for 75 of the 86 study group members whose charts were reviewed but for only 27 of the 48 control group patients with records.

Beyond recording the complaint itself, what further steps were taken by the examining physician to enable him to evaluate the patient's

90. Hospitals in which records were found for persons reporting urinary symptoms at intake, by group.

Hospital	Study group (86 persons with records)	Control group (48 persons with records)
New York Hospital	66	6
Bellevue	21	25
Metropolitan	12	16
Mount Sinai	5	9
Other	8	13

91. Basic information recorded in hospital records of persons reporting urinary symptoms at intake, by group.

Item	Study group			Control group
	NYH	Elsewhere	Total	
Urinary complaint	61/66	14/20	75/86	27/48
Prostate examined	28/31	4/7	32/38	10/17
Pelvic examination	28/35	9/13	37/48	14/31
Blood pressure	66/66	15/20	81/86	32/48
Urinalysis	66/66	15/20	81/86	30/48

complaint? Was a prostate examination performed? There were 38 males in the study group seen -- 32 of them had rectal examinations. In the control group, this examination was done on 10 out of 17 patients. Was a pelvic examination done? There were 48 women in the study group, 37 of whom had pelvic examinations, compared with 14 out of 31 in the control group. Was a blood pressure taken or urinalysis carried out at any time during the two years on this individual as far as the record shows? Blood pressures were taken on 81 out of the 86 in the study group, but on only 32 out of the 48 in the control group; and the records showed that basic information concerning the urinary tract was obtained in a considerably higher proportion of the study group, particularly for that portion of the study group who received care at the New York Hospital.

The next stage in the solution of the medical problem is diagnosis. Table 92 provides a general overview of the major diagnoses. In the study group, more benign prostatic hypertrophy was found; one might expect on the basis of chance to find about twice as much as in the control group as was actually found. It may be that more rectal examinations were done in the study group than in the control group. Pyelonephritis was diagnosed at about the same rate in both groups; maybe that illness is sufficiently symptomatic to be picked up readily under either system of care.

Perhaps the most interesting figure in Table 92 is the total number of diagnoses made. In those patients who saw a doctor, slightly more diagnoses were made in the study group (89 diagnoses in 86 patients)

92. Genito-urinary diagnoses recorded in hospital charts of persons reporting urinary symptoms at intake, by group.

| Diagnosis | Study group | | | Control group (48) |
	NYH (66)	Elsewhere (20)	Total (86)	
Urinary tract infection	14	7	21	15
Benign prostatic hypertrophy	15	0	15	5
Pyelonephritis	7	1	8	5
Diabetes	7	0	7	3
Carcinoma of urinary tract	3	1	4	1
Calculus	4	2	6	2
Other genito-urinary diagnoses	20	8	28	13
Total	70	19	89	44

than in the control group (44 diagnoses in 48 patients); patients seen at the New York Hospital were especially apt to have genito-urinary diagnoses made (70 diagnoses in 66 patients). One may at this point refer to the number of patients in each system who originally complained of urinary symptoms and compare the number of relevant diagnoses to this original base. We find that 89 diagnoses were made in 104 original study group individuals with urinary symptoms (a rate of 85 diagnoses per 100 patients), but only 44 diagnoses were made in 76 original control group individuals (a rate of 58 diagnoses per 100 patients).

After the diagnosis is made, the next stage in the solution of the problem is treatment. Table 93 shows no striking difference between study and control group in this respect. Obstruction, infection, or neoplasm were diagnosed in 39 of the 86 in the study group and in 21 of 48 in the control group. When these conditions were diagnosed, treatment was generally given in both groups.

Under both systems, follow-up seems disappointing. This is partly a failure of the patients to come in for follow-up and in some instances a failure of the system to be sufficiently persuasive. Only 37 out of the 51 patients with a genito-urinary diagnosis had a follow-up in the study group and 21 out of 27 diagnosed patients in the control group. In general, the more serious conditions tended to be followed up, whereas more minor conditions were not.

At the end of the two years, when the respondents were interviewed for the last time, they were asked about the status of the illnesses and symptoms they had originally reported on the health questionnaire. For each one originally reported, they were asked if they still had it at the time of the interview or if they had had it at any time during the past two years. Table 94 shows the results of those questions concerning "trouble urinating" and "blood in the urine."

Of 44 study group members who recalled having the symptom during the past two years, 28 reported that they still had it. Sixteen were thus

93. Proportion of cases treated among those diagnosed as needing specific treatment, by group: persons reporting urinary symptoms at intake.

| Disorder | Study group | | | Control group |
	NYH	Elsewhere	Total	
Obstruction	3/3	1/1	4/4	2/2
Infection	19/22	8/9	27/31	17/18
Neoplasm	3/3	1/1	4/4	1/1

94. Responses on the third home interview of those originally reporting urinary symptoms.

Response	"Trouble urinating"		"Blood in urine"	
	Study group	Control group	Study group	Control group
Said symptom present on original health questionnaire	104	70	20	15
Interviewed two years later	75	40	9	9
Symptom present at time of interview	28	15	1	1
Had symptom since intake but not at time of interview	16	5	3	2
Denied having symptom since intake[a]	31	20	5	6

[a]An interesting discrepancy is noted here. Seventy-five of the original 104 study group respondents reporting trouble with urination were reinterviewed. When asked whether they had trouble urinating during the past two years, only 44 out of 75 replied affirmatively. Many of those replying in the negative said they had the symptom about the time of intake into the Project but that it had cleared up promptly and had not recurred. Some denied that they had ever had urinary symptoms. Thus, the discrepancy may be due to several factors: unreliability of memory, misunderstanding of the question or the time period being asked about.

relieved of the symptom after intake. In the control group, 15 of the 20 who said they had symptoms during the past two years still had them at the time of the interview. About 37 per cent of the study group recalling the symptoms, in contrast to 25 per cent of the control group, reported clearing of symptoms during the two year period.

When the data is reviewed, it becomes apparent that a much greater proportion of study group members reporting urinary symptoms saw a physician and received a basic medical evaluation as documented in the hospital record. If this examination is regarded as good in itself, then the difference between the two systems of care is quite marked. When the frequency with which serious abnormalities are discovered and treated is examined, the advantage is seen to remain with the study group but is less striking.

In the study group, 32 of the 86 individuals receiving medical care did not have a urinary tract diagnosis made, and in the control group the proportion was even greater: 21 out of 48 persons. What does this mean? With present knowledge and techniques, a definite diagnosis cannot be established in a certain number of patients despite the most careful evaluation. This is particularly true if symptoms are minimal or intermittent. However, it is apparent that a greater proportion of control group patients had no diagnosis recorded. Of interest also is that in the study group the diagnosis tended to be made more quickly. Within the first two months after the patient came for medical care, a diagnosis was made for 36 of the 86 in the study group; in the control group, this was true of only 16 out of 48. (The difference between the two groups is statistically significant: $p<0.02$.) It can be said that study group patients who received medical care had a greater number of positive diagnoses and that diagnoses were made more quickly.

The problem of urinary tract symptoms has been followed from its inception, when the patient was aware of it, to diagnosis, treatment, follow-up, and peristence or clearing of symptoms. This method is a useful one in comparing two complex systems of medical care. As the problem was followed through various stages, it was seen that the difference between the two systems became smaller but that significant differences remained throughout. Further studies employing other symptom groups are under way.

In previous chapters the welfare population to which the Project delivered medical care, the system of medical care that the Project sought to change, and changes in behavior of the study group have been described. Responses to the Project invitation by the study group and the ways in which they subsequently used medical services as compared to the control group were examined. An important dimension of the quality of care rendered is the patient's satisfaction with it, and the satisfaction of study and control group welfare clients with the medical care they received will be analyzed below.

Method of Investigation

The 1,681 home interview respondents, speaking for the members of their respective welfare cases, are the subjects of this analysis. Because of the cooperation of the Welfare Department and the resourcefulness of the interviewers in tracking down people who had moved, NORC staff were extremely successful in locating respondents. Table 95 shows the rate of attrition of the sample for each wave of interviews. Respondents classified as "not available" were those known to have died, moved out of the five boroughs, or become institutionalized. If they are excluded, then the completion rate rises to 85 per cent for the second wave and 80 per cent for the last wave. (These are all completion rates for the attitude questionnaire, with a specific person designated as the home interview respondent. In an additional 3 to 5 per cent of cases, when the home interview respondent could not be found, some utilization data were obtained on family members from other members of the household.)

The most frequent reason for failure to obtain an interview in the other cases was inability to locate the respondent. Outright refusals were very rare: they constituted 1 per cent, 3 per cent, and 2 per cent of the first, second, and third waves respectively.

95. Completion rates for the three waves of home interviews.

Category	First wave		Second wave		Third wave	
	Number	Per cent	Number	Per cent	Number	Per cent
Interviewed	1,643	98	1,326	79	1,200	72
Not interviewed	38	2	234	15	300	20
Not available	0	–	121	6	181	8
Total	1,681	100	1,681	100	1,681	100

Patient's Awareness of the Project

One of the main objectives of the last two interviews, in addition to investigating use of medical services during the two years, was to measure patient satisfaction with the two alternative systems of care -- that offered by the Project and that provided by the existing indigent medical care system.

First, it had to be ascertained whether patients perceived the difference between the two systems. The study group members received a letter signed by the Welfare Department telling them to go to the New York Hospital if they needed medical care (and, in the A group, an appointment to the clinic). This action was crucial from the point of view of the experiment but it could well be a very small and unimportant event in the lives of some of the experimental subjects.

At the end of the third interview, when there was no danger of contaminating the research by mentioning either the New York Hospital or the Welfare Department, respondents in the study group were asked if they had received the letter of invitation. The question referred to "a letter," although in fact two letters were sent. Eighty-seven per cent replied that they had. In a population that tends to receive rather little mail, receipt of the letter, especially because it carried the authority of the Welfare Department, seems to have impressed itself on the minds of the recipients. An additional 2 per cent, who denied receiving the letter, acknowledged that they had heard of the New York Hospital Project. All these respondents, plus any others who reported attending the New York Hospital during the two years, were then asked a series of questions about the Project in order to discover how it looked to them.

One question asked if Project care was still available to the patient if he went off welfare. The precise question was: "As far as you know, could you get medical care at the New York Hospital Project during these past two years, even during periods when you might be off welfare?" The answers to this question provide further clues to why some people never responded to the invitation at all, and why others who did attend the clinic stopped coming after a while. Despite the letter of re-invitation sent in the second year to reassure patients that they were eligible for Project care even if they went off welfare, only 56 per cent of the study group knew they would still be eligible. Nineteen per cent thought they were definitely ineligible, and the remaining 25 per cent did not know one way or the other. There were differences between A and B study groups, reflecting the earlier and closer contact with the Project that the appointment method of invitation entailed. Those least likely to know they were eligible for Project care when off welfare were those who did not attend the New York Hospital at all. In this group only 42 per cent of those who could be asked realized that Project care was available to them when off welfare. (The tendency of the patient to associate medical care with being on welfare emphasizes one of the primary factors interfering with any comprehensive medical care to welfare clients, whose turnover rate is so high, See Chapter 3.)

Table 96 shows the answers to a question inquiring whether or not the Project provided certain specific services and whether or not anyone in the respondent's case had used that service during the two years. With the exception of psychiatric treatment and ambulance service, these others are services which are either unavailable or available on a very limited basis to clinic patients outside the Project. They would not be generally available, for instance, to non-Project welfare clients attending the regular clinics of the New York Hospital.

The service best known, and by far the most widely used, involved the practical matter of transportation to the clinic. Approximately three quarters of the patients who came not only knew about this service but also used it. Almost as many respondents knew that the Project would summon an ambulance when needed or pay taxi fare when a patient needed to come to a clinic or emergency room but was

96. Awareness and use of project services by study group: respondents interviewed on the third wave.

Service	Respondents who knew about service		Respondents who used service		
	Number	Per cent of those invited (N=670)	Number	Per cent of those invited (N=670)	Per cent of respondents that came (N=472)
Carfare	490	73	349	52	74
Ambulance or taxi	447	68	115	17	24
Psychiatric treatment	423	63	57	9	12
Medical advice by telephone during the day	361	54	97	14	21
Medical advice by telephone during the night	306	46	63	9	14
Doctor home visits	304	45	25	4	5
Nurse home visits	258	39	24	4	5

too ill or old or infirm to manage the bus or subway; and as many as 24 per cent of those who came received this service.

Psychiatric care on the Project was actually provided on a very limited basis -- the psychiatrist acted mainly as a consultant and could not himself treat more than a handful of patients -- but few respondents doubted that psychiatric treatment was available on the Project.

Twenty-four hour telephone coverage, through which the patients could reach a Project doctor at any hour of the day or night, was a unique feature of the Project and one that the patients seem to have appreciated and used.

Home visits were not widely made, and this fact is reflected in the patients' placing these last on the list of services they thought the Project provided.

Changes in General Attitudes

Panel questions in three general areas concerning health were asked on each of the home interviews. These related to: preferences for clinic or private doctor and, within the clinic, value placed on continuity of care with the same doctor; attitudes to doctors; images of the various hospitals known to the patients.

In analyzing changes in attitude over the three waves of interviews, study and control group respondents will be compared, with the study group subdivided into those who came and intended to stay with the Project, those who came but did not intend to return, and those who did not come. (These were the subdivisions used in describing the response to the invitation.)

Preference for Clinic or Private Doctor

At intake it was noted that as many as 40 per cent of all the respondents reported that, even if money were not a consideration, they would rather go to a clinic than a private doctor. Study and control group did not differ in this respect. Two years later, a significant difference developed between those who came to the Project and stayed with it in comparison with all the other groups (Table 97). The former increased their preference for clinic care to the extent that 69 per cent endorsed this view, compared with a slight increase to 47 per cent in all the other groups. It was not that those who responded best to the invitation were those who preferred the clinic in the first place. If anything, the reverse was true. It is suggested that the good experience with Project clinic care was the determining factor in effecting this change in attitude.

A concomitant change, occurring also in the "came and stayed" group, was an increasing value placed on continuity of care within the clinic. On the first home interview, 54 per cent of all respondents thought it very important to see the same doctor each time they went to the clinic, but 30 per cent did not think this important at all. By the last home interview, the last three groups had moved up a few percentage points in the direction of placing greater value on continuity (Table 98); but the "came and stayed" group showed a far more marked increase. Seventy-seven per cent of these respondents felt it was "very important" to see the same doctor each time they went to a

97. Changes from first (N=1,643[a]) to third (N=1,200) interview in preference for clinic care over private doctor care (in per cent).

Group	Prefer clinic at intake	Prefer clinic after two years
Study group came and stayed	38	69
Study group came and went	41	47
Study group did not come	41	47
Control group	39	47

[a]In this and the following tables, differences are not accounted for by a biased loss of respondents in the third wave. If only those interviewed on both waves are compared, the results are similar.

98. Changes from first (N=1,643) to third (N=1,200) interview in value placed by respondents on seeing the same doctor at each clinic visit (in per cent).

Group	Very important		Not important	
	First wave	Third wave	First wave	Third wave
Study group: came and stayed	56	77	27	11
Study group: came and went	55	55	33	21
Study group: did not come	52	58	33	22
Control group	55	58	29	22

clinic. It is suggested that the low value originally placed on continuity of care with the same doctor reflected a lack of the kind of experience that would breed such loyalty but that once such experience was provided, patients were ready to value continuity of care to a considerably greater extent.

On the last interview this question was followed up by asking whether or not, in fact, the respondent usually *did* see the same doctor on each clinic visit. Seventy-nine per cent of the study group who "came and stayed" replied in the affirmative, compared with 48 per cent of those who "came and went" and 22 per cent of the study group that did not come; the figure for the control group was 23 per cent. Thus it seems from the answers to these questions that those most exposed to Project care did feel that continuity, which was one of its aims, had been generally achieved and that it was appreciated.

Several questions in the last interview dealt with the subject of coordination of medical care, although they were not panel questions which had been asked on both earlier waves. One question asked if the respondent thought of any one place as the main place for him or his family to get medical care. Affirmative answers ranged from 90 per cent in the "came and stayed" group down to 64 per cent in those who came but did not stay, with the other two groups in an intermediate position. Another question asking the respondent if he thought it was a good idea to try to get *all* his medical care in one place received a similar pattern of replies, with a lesser range from 87 per cent down to 74 per cent. Again, the study group respondents who did not intend to stay with the Project were least apt to endorse the idea of centralization of care.

A final question in this section asked if the respondent had any *one* person he thought of as his own doctor. The proportion answering "yes" varied from 58 per cent of those who intended to stay with the Project, through 32 per cent of those who did not intend to stay, down to 23 per cent in the study group who did not come. In the control group, 25 per cent said they had someone they considered their own doctor.

Attitudes to Doctors

The panel question aimed at measuring general attitudes to doctors consisted of a series of items about which the respondent was asked "Do you think that is true of most doctors or not?" On the last interview, the list was read twice, once to be answered in terms of "your doctor" or "the doctors you have seen" and once in terms of "most doctors" as in the previous waves. In Table 99 is a comparison of the proportion of respondents agreeing with the statements about

99. Changes from first (*N*=1,643) to third (*N*=1,200) interview in respondents' attitudes to most doctors (in per cent).

	Study group							
	Came and stayed		Came and went		Did not come		Control group	
Attitude	First	Third	First	Third	First	Third	First	Third
They don't give you a chance to tell them exactly what your trouble is	33	38	29	37	36	40	32	40
They don't take enough personal interest in you	34	40	32	34	37	43	30	40
Doctors want you to come back for additional visits even if you don't need to	25	30	25	36	28	34	27	33
They don't tell you enough about your condition; don't explain just what the trouble is	53	51	40	46	50	55	50	51
Doctors give better care to their private patients than to their clinic patients	40	35	34	45	34	43	36	41
They tell you there's nothing wrong when you know there is	33	29	32	35	37	41	34	37
Doctors rush too much when they examine you and make you feel worse than when you came in	36	39	30	36	34	47	31	44

doctors in general on the first and third interviews. The replies are shown according to response group.

A general deterioration in attitude toward "most doctors" can be discerned in all response groups for four out of the seven critical statements that could be endorsed by respondents. (This response may also reflect a greater candor in the respondents, who were getting to know their interviewers after several visits and who were therefore more apt to "open up" and criticize more freely.) Those of the study group who "came and stayed" with the Project showed a slight improvement in attitude to "most doctors" with respect to these items: they were slightly less likely to agree on the third interview than on the first that most doctors "give better care to their private patients than to their clinic patients" or that they "tell you there's nothing wrong with you when you know there is" or that "they don't tell you enough about your condition." In all the other response groups, including the control group, respondents became more ready to criticize doctors in these three respects as well as in the other four.

When asked whether these seven statements were true of their own doctor, however, major differences between the response groups developed; these are shown in Figure 8. On six out of the seven critical items, the study group members who accepted the Project system of care were less than half as ready to criticize as any other response group. On the two positive items about doctors, used only on the last two home interviews, those accepting the Project were more than twice as ready to agree with the favorable statements about "their own doctor" than were the other groups.

Even if the two groups who came to the New York Hospital are combined -- those who intended to stay with it and those who did not -- far less criticism of doctors in this combined group is found than in either the study group members who did not come to the hospital or in the control group. Experience with the Project, then, seems to have changed patients' attitudes so far as "their own" doctor is concerned but not so much their attitudes to doctors in general.

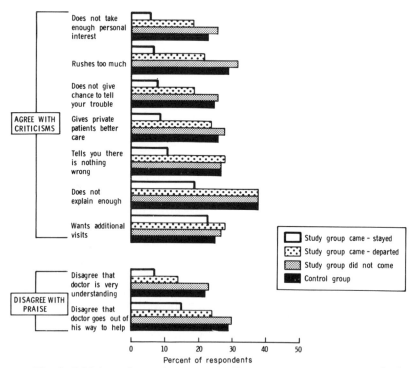

Fig. 8. Criticism of own doctor, according to response group, at end of Project

What Patients Liked and Did Not Like about the Project

In this third and final interview, Project patients were given an opportunity to express their feelings freely about the Project. Two questions asked what the respondent or his family especially liked about the Project and then what they did not like; even minor criticisms were invited. The patients followed the usual pattern of general enthusiasm for the medical care they themselves had received and reluctance to criticize it. However, in most cases their enthusiasm was so extreme that one may perhaps really believe that they found something unusually acceptable in Project care, over and above the expected positive feelings for one's own medical care. Among reasons for liking the Project, interpersonal ones headed the list, with comments such as: "You go in there and they treat you right . . . like a human being . . . You got your own doctor." Or that of an old lady of 92: "There is Dr. Z there. I remember him in my prayers -- a wonderful young doctor. He is like a close personal friend." These interpersonal reasons for liking the Project are often intertwined with comments about the high quality of medical care the patients consider they received. The old lady continued: "Everything the hospital did for me was done right because I am feeling better all the time." The first patient, after saying how he liked having his own doctor, went on: "They carry on from the last treatment. Everything seems to be the way a person should like it." He called the New York Hospital "a house of mercy, different like day and night" from the hospital he had been attending.

A young Negro with progressive muscular dystrophy also gave reasons which combined the interpersonal and medical-competence aspects of patient care: "I like the muscular therapy. It was better than here [the chronic hospital to which he was transferred]. I got more of it there. I got more attention there from the doctors and nurses and everybody was courteous, not like it is in this place . . . I got the feeling there I was going to get better. But here I don't have that feeling."

When asked for criticism, most of the respondents had none to offer. The complaints of those who did were very varied, none being particularly concentrated in any one area. The most common complaint was the distance they had to travel to reach the hospital. One patient said that what he disliked was "going up there. I was taking medication from the aftercare clinic and it slows you up -- makes you feel sleepy -- and there was complications in the traffic. You had to take the Madison Avenue bus and walk all the way over to Lexington. Complications in traveling."

The second most common complaint was the length of time one had to wait in clinic. As one patient put it: "I suppose everybody complains about the waiting and you've got your share of it at the New York

Hospital as any other place. But I wouldn't make a production out of a complaint like this. It's just that hospital waiting is always somehow annoying. Maybe it's because there's a bit of anxiety attached to it and it's really not just relaxed waiting but a special kind of waiting of people who don't feel so good." Several complained that full dental care was not available; one, for instance, reported: "Dental clinic. They gave me an appointment. The doctor sent me to see if I could have my tooth done and they told me not to go back unless I have pain." A few patients had serious complaints which explained their definite rejection of Project care after initially responding to the invitation; but these were a small minority.

Because it it easy to elicit expressions of satisfaction and difficult to evoke criticism of a patient's own experience with doctors and hospitals, reliance was not put solely on the answers to these two questions in measuring satisfaction with the Project. A much more sensitive measure would seem to be the question that asked of all respondents, study and control group, and out of the context of any discussion of a particular hospital: "Altogether, would you say the medical care you (your family) got this past year was better, about the same, or worse than the medical care you got the year before?" The question was asked on both the second and third home interviews; but because the great majority of patients came in the first year, the replies on the second wave are shown here (Table 100).

Few respondents in either group said their care was worse in the past year than in the preceding one; but significantly more of the study group than the control group rated their care as better. To see if this was related to their experience on the Project, Table 101 shows the hospitals used by study group cases in relation to rating of medical care. This table does indeed show that those who used the New York Hospital were more likely to rate their care as better; those who used it exclusively were even more apt to do so than those who used it together with other hospitals.

100. Rating of first year's medical care compared with year before Project, by study and control groups (N=1,326 second-wave respondents).

Medical care	Study group		Control group	
	Number	Per cent	Number	Per cent
Better	293	36	108	21
Same	410	51	312	60
Worse	29	4	26	5
Don't know or no answer	77	7	71	14
Total	809	100	517	100

101. Rating of first year's medical care compared with year before Project, study group only, by hospitals used (N=809 second wave study group respondents).

Hospital	Better		Same		Worse		DK or NA		Total	
	Number	Per cent	Number	Per cent	Number	Per cent	Number	Per cent	Number	Per cent
NYH only	129	55	82	35	8	3	14	6	233	100
NYH and other(s)	105	49	93	43	9	4	9	4	216	100
Other(s) only	55	19	209	70	11	4	21	7	296	100
No hospital used	4	6	26	41	1	1	33	52	64	100
Total	293	36	410	51	29	4	77	7	809	100

Hospital Image

At each interview a series of statements descriptive of hospitals was read off to respondents and they were asked to name those hospitals in New York City which seemed to fit each statement. They could name more than one hospital if they wished. Table 102 shows the "attitudes to" or "opinions about" the four major hospitals at intake. Study and control groups are combined here because there was no reason to expect differences in initial attitudes between these randomly selected groups.

As in the selection of hospitals that were "best liked" and "least liked" (see Chapter 4), the New York Hospital is not very often mentioned; but when it is, it is almost always in a favorable light. Bellevue is mentioned far more than any other, with a mixed image that balances "has the best doctors" against "overcrowded" and "friendly" against "keeps you waiting." Metropolitan comes next in frequency of mention, with a greater weighting of negative items. Mount Sinai has mostly favorable mentions, the chief criticism being that it is "only for the rich." "All other hospitals" include a large number of different ones, close to a hundred, with no particular one mentioned nearly as often as the four leading hospitals. A great many of the negative attributes evoked mention of some of these other hospitals, rather than the leading four.

As changes in hospital image were observed over the study period, answers were sought to the following questions: What impact did the Project have on awareness of the New York Hospital (in terms of the number of times it is mentioned)? Did the image of the New York Hospital change, and, if so, was the change different for the different response groups? Did those who came start out with a different image of the New York Hospital? What was the effect of the Project on the study group's attitude to the other three main hospitals? For this analysis, as with the other attitude questions, the study group was divided into those who came and intended to stay with the Project, those who came but did not intend to continue there, and those who did not come. These three were compared with the control group.

Awareness of the New York Hospital. All three sub-divisions of the study group showed a greatly increased awareness of the New York Hospital at the end of the study compared with the beginning. (Table 103). To make comparisons easier, this table has been converted into rates per thousand respondents. As might be expected, there were differences between the three sub-groups. Those who came and stayed with the Project were almost 5 times as likely to mention the New York Hospital in response to the list of attributes on the third interview as on the first. It is interesting to find an almost equally great increase in

102. Number of times the four leading hospitals were mentioned on first interview, in response to list of attributes (N=1,643).

Response	NYH Number	Per cent	Bellevue Number	Per cent	Metropolitan Number	Per cent	Mt. Sinai Number	Per cent	All Others
Easy to get to	106	18	784	21	421	23	221	21	529
Good but too far away	117	20	123	4	59	3	111	10	1,288
Has the best doctors	129	22	543	16	89	5	208	19	799
Friendly	121	20	399	12	213	12	190	18	857
Only for rich people	70	12	5	—a	8	—	134	12	1,469
Keeps you waiting far too long	23	4	465	14	301	16	96	9	818
Overcrowded	10	2	554	16	372	20	79	7	738
Not enough doctors and nurses	7	1	193	6	166	9	29	3	1,280
Gloomy or dirty	1	—	226	7	94	5	3	—	1,360
Doesn't treat you like a person	6	1	135	4	136	7	12	1	1,375
Total Responses	590	100	3,367	100	1,859	100	1,083	100	10,513

a Less than 1 per cent.

103. Changes from first to third interview in rate of mention of four leading hospitals (rate per 1,000).

Group	NYH		Bellevue		Metropolitan		Mt. Sinai	
	First	Third	First	Third	First	Third	First	Third
Study group: came and stayed	557	2,710	1,933	1,635	1,181	1,157	579	453
Study group: came and went	384	1,516	1,969	1,611	1,111	1,053	636	663
Study group: didn't come	157	388	2,201	2,140	1,195	1,198	789	782
Control group	340	434	1,978	1,952	1,190	1,217	689	756

awareness in those who came to the New York Hospital but did not stay: they mentioned it nearly four times as often on the third wave as on the first. Those who did not come showed a twofold increase. In the control group, on the other hand, there are only chance fluctuations in the mentions of any of the four hospitals from first to third wave.

Tendency to mention the New York Hospital on the first interview is related to response to the subsequent invitation: those who came, especially those who stayed with the Project, were far more likely to have mentioned it than those who later did not respond to the invitation.

Mentions of the other three leading hospitals do not seem to have been affected in the study group members who had no contact with the Project. In both sub-groups who came to the Project (those who intended to stay and those who did not) there was less tendency to mention Bellevue on the third wave, but no difference with respect to Metropolitan or Mount Sinai.

Change in Image of the New York Hospital. With respect to the characteristics attributed to the New York Hospital by the various response groups before and after experience with the Project (Table 103), it is evident that there was to a limited extent a selective mechanism at work in determining which patients would respond to the invitation. Those who came for care, whether they stayed or not, were more likely to start by thinking it accessible, rather than "good but too far away." (The simple explanation for many would be that they *did* live nearer it, but some patients living about equidistant from two hospitals sometimes perceived their accessibility differently.) And those who subsequently came and stayed with the Project did have a somewhat more favorable view of the hospital at intake than the others in the study group. But the differences were not large. For those who did not come at all, it does not seem to have been an unfavorable image of the New York Hospital that kept many of them away.

The third wave responses show that there is a vastly increased number in the study group who now mention the New York Hospital, and that its good image seems generally to persist. For those who came and stayed with the Project, the New York Hospital is now mentioned even more frequently than Bellevue or Metropolitan and generally in a much more favorable light. Its overriding characteristics are thought to be its "friendliness" (31 per cent of all mentions) and that it "has the best doctors" (26 per cent of all mentions). This extremely positive view of the hospital could perhaps have been predicted in those who decided to stay with it. A less expected finding, perhaps, is the extremely favorable image of the hospital held by those who came to the Project but did not stay. Proportionally almost as many consider that it is "friendly" and "has the best doctors" as among those who did stay. Those who say the New York Hospital is "good but too far away" seem to provide the main reason for not staying with the Project. Those of the study group who did not come are the most likely to consider it inaccessible. They are no more likely, in general, to criticize the hospital on the third wave than they were at the first interview.

Attitudes to Other Hospitals. The attitudes to Bellevue, Metropolitan, and Mount Sinai before and after the study are shown in Appendix Tables A-41, A-42, and A-43. In general, there is no consistent difference in initial attitude to these three hospitals to correlate with the subsequent response of the study group to the New York Hospital; those who later responded completely, partially, or not at all to the invitation to switch their medical care to the New York Hospital started out with broadly similar attitudes to the three other hospitals in the neighborhood.

A look at the third wave of interviews indicates that there is a general tendency (seen also in the control group's attitude to the New York Hospital) to rate fewer hospitals as "easy to get to" and more as "good but too far away." This reflects the fact that the welfare recipients, originally all living in the Yorkville district between 6th and 106th Streets on the east side of Manhattan, gradually scattered during the two years -- many moving to other parts of Manhattan and some to other boroughs.

Otherwise, there seem to be only random variations in attitudes among respondents in the control group and the study group who did not try the Project. In the study group who "came and stayed," on the other hand, their favorable view of the New York Hospital was accompanied by a less positive view of the other hospitals, especially of Bellevue and Metropolitan. In the "came and went" group, the opinion of other hospitals on the third wave was mixed.

This analysis has examined the attitudes to hospitals of whole groups or sub-groups, for instance, of *all* those in the study group who came to the Project and were available for interview on the first wave, compared with *all* those in this sub-group who were available for the third wave interview. A more detailed analysis is planned later of only those who were interviewed on both waves. The attitude change or persistence in individual respondents, as well as the aggregate opinions of the same group of respondents, can then be examined.

104. Attitude to New York Hospital, before and after Project, by response group.

	Study Group											
	Came and Stayed				Came and Went				Didn't Come			
	Before		After		Before		After		Before		After	
Items endorsed	Number	Per cent	Number	Per cent	Number	Per cent	Number	Per cent	Number	Per cent	Number	Per cent
Easy to get to	42	19	139	14	7	18	9	6	4	8	4	4
Good, but to far away	36	16	197	19	8	21	42	29	17	36	41	44
Only for rich people	19	8	43	4	8	21	12	9	12	24	12	13
Has the best doctors	52	23	260	26	5	14	30	21	7	14	20	21
Friendly	58	26	319	32	7	18	38	26	6	12	14	15
Keeps you waiting much too long	8	4	33	3	2	5	7	5	2	4	1	1
Overcrowded	4	2	13	1	0	0	2	1	1	2	1	1
Not enough doctors and nurses	3	1	7	1	0	0	0	0	0	0	0	0
Gloomy or dirty	0	0	2	—a	0	0	1	1	0	0	1	1
Doesn't treat you like a person	3	1	3	—	1	3	3	2	0	0	0	0
Total responses	225	100	1,016	100	38	100	144	100	49	100	94	100
Persons interviewed	404		375		99		95		313		242	

aLess than 1 per cent.

104 (Continued)

Items endorsed	Control Group			
	Before		After	
	Number	Per cent	Number	Per cent
Easy to get to	38	18	26	13
Good, but to far away far away	40	19	46	23
Only for rich people	27	12	25	13
Has the best doctors	51	24	52	26
Friendly	38	18	37	18
Keeps you waiting much too long	9	4	8	4
Overcrowded	4	2	6	3
Not enough doctors and nurses	4	2	0	0
Gloomy or dirty	0	0	0	0
Doesn't treat you like a person	2	1	1	—
Total responses	213	100	201	100
Persons interviewed	636		463	

15 | Summary and Conclusion

The New York Hospital—Cornell Project, 1960—1965, was an experiment in the organization of medical care services. Its purpose was to determine the feasibility of a voluntary teaching hospital serving as a base to provide complete medical care to a population of welfare recipients and to study the utilization, cost, and quality of that care. The Project evolved in response to the determination of the New York City Department of Health and Welfare to improve the quality and lessen the fragmentation of the medical care available to welfare clients.

The Existing Medical Care System

The medical care system for the poor as it existed in New York City at the start of the Project was highly fragmented and often interfered with continuity of patient care. Indigent New Yorkers received the bulk of their medical care in the clinics, emergency rooms, and wards of municipal hospitals; city hospitals also provided short term psychiatric hospitalization, limited psychiatric clinic care, and hospital-based home care. In many instances patients moving a few blocks would change districts and therefore had to change municipal hospitals. Voluntary hospitals provided similar medical services but were used less than the city hospitals by truly indigent patients. The Department of Health ran well-baby clinics (sick children were referred elsewhere, but hospital pediatric clinics often would not see them when they were well), dental clinics for children up to twelve years, chest clinics for tuberculosis, venereal disease clinics, and some diagnostic, coronary, obesity, and health maintenance clinics. Some dental care was provided by the school health service in school clinics and by private sources. Long-term mental hospitalization and some psychiatric aftercare were handled by the state, and limited psychiatric care was given under other auspices. The Department of Welfare provided -- to those on welfare - panel physician home visits, dental clinics, eye clinics, and dentures, eyeglasses, and other medical appliances; it paid for visiting nurse service, homemaker service, nursing home care, out-patient care at voluntary hospitals, transportation to the clinics, and drugs prescribed by panel physicians. Coordination of this care was by and large left up to the patient.

The New York Hospital—Cornell Project

In place of this fragmentary system, the New York Hospital—Cornell Project offered a full range of services under the auspices of one institution. For the purpose of the experiment, the hospital agreed to invite about one thousand welfare cases. The thousand cases were to be selected from newly registered welfare recipients in the local welfare district. From July 1, 1961, through June 30, 1962, all those accepted on welfare in the Yorkville welfare district were interviewed by Project staff. Sixty per cent of the cases were randomly allocated into the study group and invited to receive all their needed medical care at the New York Hospital. The remaining 40 per cent, the control group, were left to obtain their medical care under the existing system. Both the study and control groups were followed for two years.

Chart Study

Before the experiment began, a study of the records kept by the Welfare Department on 374 clients newly registered in the Yorkville welfare district in 1959 was carried out. This study showed that in a cohort of cases newly accepted on welfare, less than half would be on welfare two years later, and less than a quarter would be on continuously. Cases with dependent children tend to close and reopen, often at very brief intervals. Some people, especially among the unemployed, receive assistance briefly and are not on welfare again during a two year period, whereas others of the unemployed have physical or psychological impairment that leads them eventually to be reclassified as disabled. Even among the aging many cases are closed within a two year period, only some by death. However, virtually all those removed from welfare rolls during the two years of Project observation would still be medically indigent. It was therefore decided to provide the same services for the full two years of the Project to all persons invited, whether or not they remained on welfare during that time.

Feasibility

Allocation of space for the Project and recruitment of staff at the hospital were readily accomplished. The services offered included complete medical and pediatric care, including social casework, public health nursing, and psychiatric consultation and treatment. Ambulant, emergency, and bed care in hospital, home, and nursing home were provided or coordinated by Project staff. A complete medical history and physical examination were given, usually on the first visit. Appropriate tests were made as care began. Well-child care and extensions of normal eye and dental clinic service were provided. Disability evaluations were made for the Welfare Department. Every adult patient was assigned a personal staff physician to insure continuity of care. The three pediatricians worked as an intercommunicating team, so that each of them came to know all the families.

Communication among members of the clinical team was emphasized. Direct-line telephones were established and daily written forms exchanged between medicine and pediatrics. Weekly staff meetings and annual chart reviews systematically reviewed the patient load, and frequent conferences were held on individual patients and families. Patients lost to follow-up were given three more appointments, and if seriously in need of care were then pursued by home visit or through welfare or visiting nurse service. Social casework nearly always involved working with the Welfare Department and a third of the time with other social agencies as well. Casework service was also extended to nursing home patients and their families.

Services not offered directly by the New York Hospital included restorative dentistry, chronic hospitalization, mental hospitalization, and some psychiatric clinic care. For patients who needed such services, Project staff tried to refer them to appropriate facilities, follow their progress, and resume contact when those referral services ended.

Project nurses were responsible for much of the day-to-day coordination. They gave direct patient service and called on the regular general medical and pediatric clinic nursing staffs when needed. The nursing coordinator introduced and interpreted the Project to nurses throughout the hospital, to the Health Department Bureau of Nursing, and to the personnel of nursing homes. She also acted as liaison agent with other hospitals and clinics and, together with other regular staff nurses, coordinated the patients' care through all the various facilities with which they became involved, keeping the Project physicians informed about their assigned patients' activities.

From their intimate knowledge of the patients, the nurses also assisted in annual medical chart reviews and in the research. They had access to the welfare data as well as to the Project research records. In the clinics they devoted much of their time to problem patients, made referrals to dental care and podiatry, and supervised the delivery of eyeglasses. In their constant availability to patients and the extensive role they played in patient care, the Project nurses combined the responsibilities of office nurse, clinic nurse, and public health nurse.

The bilingual (English and Spanish) clinic clerks who, under supervision of the nursing staff, handled appointments, answered telephones, filled out welfare forms, and disbursed carfare knew patients so well that months and sometimes years later they could supply the research staff with a detail on a particular patient or family without referring to their records. Their relationship with patients was one of the most important aspects of their jobs and provided much of the Project's continuity and coordination.

Response to the Invitation

There were 1,029 welfare cases (2,504 persons) in the study group. The single most important factor determining whether or not these persons would come to the New York Hospital for care was found to be the way they were invited. All study group patients were told in a letter from the Welfare Department to go to the New York Hospital when they needed medical care, and a brochure on a New York Hospital letterhead supplied details on how to obtain the various medical services provided. Half the study group cases (the appointment group) were sent appointments for a physical examination along with the letter of invitation to the New York Hospital. The other half (the demand group) received only the invitation and were left to come when they saw the need. Two years later, one or more persons had come to the New York Hospital from 74 per cent of the cases in the appointment group, and one or more persons from only 51 per cent of the cases in the demand group responded. The total study group response was 63 per cent of the 1,029 study group cases.

Other factors determining response were address, age, ethnic group, welfare category, current use of other medical facilities, and familiarity with the New York Hospital. The Yorkville welfare district extended at that time along Manhattan's East Side from 6th Street to 106th Street -- a long narrow strip with the New York Hospital situated in the wealthy middle section and four fifths of the Project welfare population in slum areas at either end. Two city hospitals, Bellevue to the south and Metropolitan to the north (along with Mount Sinai, a voluntary hospital) were much closer to that welfare population and had served most of them in the past. People most likely to come to the New York Hospital were the aged and disabled white native American and European-born living reasonably close to the New York Hospital and often familiar with it. People least likely to come (especially when the letter of invitation did *not* include an appointment) were the Puerto Rican families living far from the hospital, unfamiliar with it, and currently using Bellevue or Metropolitan hospitals. Families often had to face transporting all the children to the hospital when one of them or the parent was in need of medical care; and Puerto Ricans, who made up 55 per cent of the Project population, were sometimes particularly reluctant to face the confusion of an unfamiliar hospital when they had a language problem.

Two more factors affecting response were the frequency with which the poor change their dwellings and the turnover of the welfare case-load. Frequent moves made it hard for the clinical staff to keep in touch with Project patients, especially when they had moved out of Manhattan. Many, as anticipated, were not on welfare for long, and 19 per cent of all respondents mistakenly thought they could not get Project care when they were off welfare, with another 25 per cent uncertain if they could. If they moved to another welfare district, a new investigator might make other arrangements for medical care. Furthermore, disabilities made travel to the clinic difficult for some, a few never got the invitation, others were too disturbed or retarded to comprehend it, and the existing system, particularly the city ambulance service, took some patients to other facilities against their will.

Patients responded well to the invitation, considering the difficulties of distance and disability that faced them. Sending a specific appointment to half the study group brought out the importance of this method to improve patient attendance and response. Once they made contact with the hospital, most of the patients stayed with the Project and brought other family members. After two years, those available for questioning were more than 9 to 2 in favor of staying with this source of medical care.

Health Status of the Study Population

Although from questionnaire responses the population studied did not seem especially prone to seek medical care, they reported at intake to welfare many illnesses and symptoms. As checked by Project physicians, the amount of reported illness was not exaggerated. Adult patients had much organic disease, a far higher rate than was found in an urban population such as that of the Baltimore survey.[1] They also had an especially high rate of psychiatric illness as compared with other studies and with the urban population in general. In each of the two years of observation about 25 per cent of the adults attending the Project clinic at the New York Hospital were hospitalized there. Social factors contributing to illness, such as housing, family, and work problems, were common.

Almost two thirds of the children were found to have health problems at the time they first came to the Project, and for one out of seven it was a serious condition. Few children were considered to have had adequate previous care. Ninety-five per cent had one or more diagnoses made during their two years on the Project, with acute respiratory disease heading the list of illness. Parasitic disease, tuberculosis, and anemia were other important problems. Psychiatric diagnoses were also prominent, with "behavioral disorders" the most frequently listed. Social factors were implicated in the health status of two fifths of all pediatric patients. Taking adults and children together, 51 per cent of the families and individuals seen were referred to social service.

1. Commission on Chronic Illness, *Chronic Illness in a Large City: The Baltimore Survey*, IV, *Chronic Illness in the United States* (Cambridge, Mass.: Harvard University Press, 1957).

Experience with Study Group Patients

Four Project internists cared for the adult patients. They spent a combined average of 46 three-hour sessions a month and averaged 3.5 patient visits per doctor per session, including new and revisit patients. The three Project pediatricians averaged 29.3 three-hour sessions a month with 4.4 patient visits per doctor per session. More walk-in visits were made to pediatrics (one quarter of all visits) than to medicine (less than one eighth of the visits). The half-time psychiatrist spent most of his time seeing patients on referral from other staff members, in order to determine disability, advise on referral to community agencies, and render short-term therapy. About a quarter of his time was spent in individual and group consultation with staff members.

About half of all the adult visits in the first year were made to the Project physicians; nearly all the others were to specialty clinics, with only 4 per cent to the emergency room. Referrals for specialty care were most frequently made to eye, dental, surgery, and ear, nose, and throat clinics, in that order. The orthopedist was the most frequent "on the spot" consultant, followed by the surgeon, dermatologist, and gynecologist. Seventy per cent of the childrens' visits in the first year were to Project pediatricians, 14 per cent to specialty clinics, 8 per cent to the emergency room, and 5 per cent were home doctor visits.

Most people came within three months of receiving the invitation. The number of demand group adults and children reached a peak in the very first month; for the appointment group the peak came in the second month, because appointments were spaced to avoid overloading the clinic. The Welfare Department referred 144 adults for disability evaluation in the first year, and because they had to be done within a short time span, they contributed markedly to the congestion of adult patients in the early months. In pediatrics, the patient load built up more slowly than in medicine, with a considerable number of children coming for the first time in the second year. Two thirds of the adults were designated as still active in the clinic after one year, and nearly half after two years.

Proportion of Care Given by the Project

Even though the Project offered a relatively full range of medical services, those who came did receive some care outside the Project. Coordination was most successful with ambulant care, less so with hospitalization. Those of the study group who came to the New York Hospital obtained the great majority of their ambulatory care from or through the Project. When these people went elsewhere, it was usually before or after coming to the New York Hospital, seldom concurrently.

However, they were in-patients at other hospitals quite often. This was sometimes because they needed care not available through the New York Hospital, such as psychiatric hospitalization or general admissions over sixty days. But it was often because the city ambulance, despite their requests to be taken to the New York Hospital, took them to the hospital for the district in which they lived or in which they were taken ill.

Comparisons of Study and Control Groups

An attempt was made to measure and compare the total use of medical services anywhere in or near New York City by the appointment study group, the demand study group, and the control group during the two years. Three waves of home interviews by the National Opinion Research Center, conducted at intake and one and two years later, asked about sources and amount of medical care used; these reports were checked against the hospital records in a subsample of cases.

Comparing the whole of the appointment study group, demand study group, and control group, total doctor visits per 1,000 persons at risk were 8.1, 7.1, and 6.5 respectively in the first year; in the second year they were 5.5, 5.2, and 4.5.

In the entire appointment study group, including those who came to the New York Hospital and those who did not, about 60 per cent of this care was provided by or through the Project in the first year and about 65 per cent in the second year. If one considers only those members of the appointment group who came to the New York Hospital, then the proportion of ambulant care they received there rises to about 76 per cent in the first year and about 80 per cent in the second.

For the demand study group (those invited to the New York Hospital but left to initiate care there when they felt the need), services provided by the Project constituted about 40 per cent of the entire group's ambulant care in the first year; the proportion remained unchanged in the second year. For those of the demand study group who came to the New York Hospital, the Project provided almost as high a proportion of their doctor visits as it did for the appointment study group, that is, nearly 75 per cent in each year.

By and large, study group members who did not come to the Project were low utilizers; they averaged far fewer visits than those who came and fewer than the average member of the control group.

The national average for general hospitalization in 1962 was slightly below one day per person (that is, 905 days per 1,000 persons). This rate was greatly exceeded by both study groups and by the control group, with rates per 1,000 persons of 2,610 days for the appointment group, 2,838 for the demand group, and 2,467 for the control group in the first year. By the second year the rates had dropped to 1,799, 2,532, and 1,510 respectively. In all three groups it was the excessively long stays that contributed most to this surplus. The admission rate (national average 132 per 1,000) was exceeded by both study groups in both years, and by the control group in the first year only. (The admission rates per 1,000 for the appointment group, the demand group, and the control group for the first year were 201, 210, and 170 respectively. Second year admissions, listed in the same group order, were 149, 151, and 102.) This pattern for the control group in the second year--of a lower than average hospital admission rate but a far higher than average length of stay -- may indicate a relative inaccessibility of medical care to the indigent in the existing system, especially as short-term welfare recipients go off relief. Length of stay declined in the second year in the appointment group only. The continued high number of hospital days in the demand group was due in part to a disproportionate number of very long admissions, for which there is no ready explanation.

A comparison of chronic care, including admissions to state mental hospitals, chronic hospitals, nursing homes, and home care, showed more admissions and days for the appointment group than for the demand group. The control group had considerably fewer admissions than either study group, suggesting that additional referrals to long-term care were prompted by Project care.

Cost of Care

A major question related to feasibility is that of costs. Two approaches were used, one a careful audit of costs at the New York Hospital and the other an analysis of estimated costs of the care obtained anywhere in the city by the control group as compared with the study group. Using the first approach -- audit of the cost of the care provided to members of the study group at the New York Hospital -- the average cost per person eligible for care was $99 for the first year and $79 for the second year; for those actually served it was $240 per patient for the first year and $218 for the second.

The estimated cost comparison of study and control groups, which included care given from all sources, showed that the study group patients averaged $254 per person eligible for care in the first year and $241 in the second year, compared with $185 for the controls in the first year and $143 in the second year. Total estimated cost per person was no higher for the appointment study group than for the demand group.

Coordinated care for welfare clients with their considerable amount of illness was thus more expensive under the experimental system than under the existing system.

Quality and Effectiveness of Care

In comparing the effectiveness of study and control group systems of welfare medical care, the most crucial problem was the relatively short period of observation (two years) in view of the chronic, long-term character of most of the serious medical problems encountered. Studies of mortality, both infant and adult, did not significantly differentiate the systems. The overall death rate of the study and control groups combined was 13.4 per thousand, which is slightly higher than the rate for New York City (11.4) for a similar period. In the age group 30-69, however, the Project rates, combining both study and control groups, were two and a half times that of the city. The causes of death in both groups combined followed a pattern similar to that of the general population except that the higher incidence of tuberculosis made respiratory disease the fourth leading cause of death, with accidents, including suicide, close behind. (A rank order listing of the causes of death for Project patients can be found in Table 81.) In deaths occurring at home the proportion referred to the medical examiner was higher than in the city in general.

Comparison of study and control group perinatal care in the first year showed little systematic difference between the groups as a whole. Mothers coming to the New York Hospital to have their babies, however, were more likely to return for post-partum and other health care than other study group mothers, or than control group mothers. They were also far more likely to bring their babies for well-child care at the hospital where they were delivered. The difficulty of reaching young families, who generally lived at the far ends of the Yorkville welfare district, is reflected in the fact that only one-third of the study group babies were born at the New York Hospital in the first year.

Another approach to comparison of the effectiveness of the two systems of care was devised by regarding medical care as a problem-solving activity with the following seven stages: recognition by the patient of the existence of a medical problem; availability and use of help by the patient; identification and recognition of the signs and symptoms by the physican; categorization of the problem (diagnosis); action on the problem (treatment); resolution of the problem (cure or rehabilitation); and follow-up.

This method of studying medical care effectiveness started with an analysis of those patients who complained in the baseline health questionnaire of "trouble with urination" or "blood in the urine" (104 study group and 76 control patients). Significant differences between the two systems were shown at most stages of the process. The most important difference was the greater proportion of study group patients who received medical care for these symptoms. There was also a significantly higher proportion of diagnoses made in the study group that required definitive medical or surgical therapy. Finally, more of the study patients stated in the final health questionnaire that their symptoms had cleared during the two year period.

Patient Satisfaction

The most distinct difference between study and control groups showed in the patients' satisfaction with their medical care. The three waves of home interviews monitored changes in attitudes to doctors, hospitals, and medical care in general and asked specific questions about satisfaction with care received in the year prior to interview. Patients using the New York Hospital in the first year, especially those using it exclusively, were much more likely than others to rate their year's medical care as "better" than that of the previous year. When questioned directly, patients evinced enthusiasm for Project care, and few criticized it. Most frequent criticisms were of the difficulty of getting to the New York Hospital and of waiting time.

The general attitudes of those who came to the Project and especially of those who intended to stay with it changed in the following ways: they were more likely after two years to prefer clinic care to private care; they were more apt to value continuity of care in the clinic and especially to consider that they did experience continuity of doctor care; they were more likely to feel that they had a "main source" for their medical care; more felt that there was someone they considered to be their "own" doctor.

The patients had a good understanding of present-day complexities of medical care and apparently appreciated a genuine attempt to personalize and coordinate it.

Conclusion

The New York Hospital–Cornell Project established that a voluntary teaching hospital could render a full range of medical services in a personalized and coordinated way to a population of welfare recipients in the community. The relative success of the undertaking depended on a number of innovations in customary out-patient practice. The most important of these were: (1) providing a clinical team within the hospital that could come to know the patients over a span of years and that would provide the continuity such care requires; (2) taking responsibility for the care of people in the community before they presented themselves for treatment (taking the initiative in beginning care, with an appointment for a physical examination, proved even more successful than leaving the patient to establish contact himself); (3) guaranteeing availability of services to patients so that they did not face repeated screening for eligibility.

For future programs some means is needed for continuity of financing for patients who go on and off welfare. Medicaid may take care of this problem. Prepayment is also desirable if use of preventive services is to be fostered.

When a whole medical care system is studied rather than, as is more often the case, the care provided by a particular institution, it becomes apparent that many factors in the medical environment of the indigent still militate against coordination of their care. The Project staff found most of the welfare clients they served and studied to be people who were unexpectedly knowledgeable about the advantages and drawbacks of the various medical facilities available to them. They were making efforts to coordinate their own care -- the clinic shopper was a rarity -- but constantly came up against barriers like eligibility requirements and districting rules. When these were removed, as in the care given by the Project, patients tended to stay with such a system once they had made contact with it and seemed most appreciative of continuous, personalized medical care.

Welfare clients were found to have many illnesses, and from the experience with the Project, they seemed to be particularly vulnerable when first registering for public assistance. It might be desirable as a general rule, therefore, to give new welfare clients appointments for a complete medical examination as soon as registration is completed.

Access to providers of medical care is a particular problem for the indigent, and it is important to reduce the barriers to access as much as possible if these patients are to make optimal use of health services. Distance from the source was found to be a major factor in the Project, as has been noted, and community planning should therefore include attention to provision of facilities within easy reach of the population to be served. Districting may make continuity of care difficult, however, and some flexibility should be permitted to allow patients to continue to use customary sources of care.

Comprehensive, hospital-based care was found to be relatively expensive, and it was difficult to relate the extra cost to improvement in the usual measures of mortality and morbidity. The length of the observation period may well have been too short to detect significant differences between study and control groups, given the state of ill health of the welfare population. Beginning a new program is also more expensive than is routine provision of care once the program has been established. It seems likely that as more experience is accumulated with comprehensive care programs for the indigent they will be found to be less expensive in the long run and that their effectiveness in improving the health of the population served may be demonstrated over a time span longer than could be observed in the New York Hospital–Cornell Project. Moreover, apart from the proof of cost effectiveness, medical care must be thought of in terms of meeting the demands of patients for comfort and support. There can be little question that the Project met these requirements for the patients who made use of it. The effort to extend such care to far greater numbers is the next challenge.

Appendices

Index

Appendix A

Supplementary Tables (A-1 to A-43)

A-1. New admissions to welfare in New York City, July 1961.

Category	Number of cases	Per cent of cases
Aid to Dependent Children	1,789	33
Old Age Assistance	667	12
Aid to the Disabled	814	15
Aid to the Blind	28	
Home Relief	1,512	28
Temporary Aid to Dependent Children	645	12
Total[a]	5,455	100

[a]MAA is omitted because it only started in April–May 1961, and the large number of new admissions in the early months distorted the usual picture.

A-2. Comparability of A, B, and C groups on selected variables.

Variable	Result of significance test
Average age	No significant difference
Proportion over or under 60	No significant difference
Sex	No significant difference
Single or family case	No significant difference
Ethnic group	Significantly more Puerto Ricans in control group
Welfare category	Significantly more PAD's in study group

A-3. Project population by welfare category at intake.

Category	Cases Number	Cases Per cent	Persons Number	Persons Per cent
Aid to Dependent Children	592	35	2,157	52
Temporary Aid to Dependent Children	146	9	747	18
Home Relief—family cases	95	6	437	10
Total Family Cases	833	50	3,341	80
Pending Aid to the Disabled	233	14	233	6
Aid to the Disabled	60	3	60	1
Aid to the Blind	12	1	12	a
Old Age Assistance	236	14	236	6
Medical Aid to the Aged	52	3	52	1
Home Relief—single cases	255	15	255	6
Total single cases	848	50	848	20
Total	1,681	100	4,189	100

[a]Less than 1 per cent.

A-4. Project population by ethnic group and welfare category (total persons).

Welfare category at intake	Puerto Rican		Negro		Non-Puerto Rican white		Total persons	
	Number	Per cent	Number	Per cent	Number	Per cent	Number	Per cent
Old Age Assistance, Medical Aid to Aged	28	10	13	5	247	86	288	100
Aid to Disabled, Pending Aid to Disabled, Aid to the Blind	68	22	46	15	191	63	305	100
Home Relief (single)	91	36	38	15	126	49	255	100
Total single case-members	187	22	97	11	564	67	848	100
Aid to Dependent Children	1,311	61	433	20	413	19	2,157	100
Temporary Aid to Dependent Children	531	71	154	21	62	8	747	100
Home Relief (family)	290	66	55	13	92	19	437	100
Total family case-members	2,132	64	642	19	567	17	3,341	100
Total persons	2,319	55	739	18	1,131	27	4,189	100

A-5. Project population by ethnic group, single or family case-membership, and address at intake (total persons).

Address at intake	Puerto Rican			Negro			Non-Puerto Rican white			Total persons		
	Single	Family	Total	Single	Family	Total	Single	Family	Total	Single	Family	Total
6th–13th Street	54	977	1,031	16	129	145	127	141	268	197	1,247	1,444
14th–29th Street	39	212	251	12	18	30	136	80	216	187	310	497
30th–56th Street	5	24	29	2	10	12	66	52	118	73	86	159
57th–95th Street	8	76	84	4	13	17	202	197	399	214	286	500
96th–106th Street	81	843	924	63	472	535	33	97	130	177	1,412	1,589
Total persons	187	3,132	2,319	97	642	739	564	567	1,131	848	3,341	4,189

A-6. Past and present illnesses reported by adults at intake (N=1,980).

Illnesses[a]	Has now	Has had but not now	Total Number	Per cent
Suffer from nerves	891	41	932	47
Sinus trouble	259	105	364	18
Hypertension	204	149	353	18
Arthritis	286	39	325	16
Varicose veins	268	55	323	16
Allergies	215	92	307	16
Severe anemia	97	188	285	14
Women's trouble (ovary or womb)	78	206	284	14
Hemorrhoids	99	162	261	13
Heart trouble	198	53	251	13
Kidney or bladder disease	96	125	221	11
Asthma	137	79	216	11
Tumor	24	177	201	10
Parasites or worms	13	186	199	10
Hernia	60	130	190	10
Serious lung trouble[b]	68	120	188	10
Rheumatic fever	17	84	101	5
Tuberculosis	26	71	97	5
Gallstones	12	82	94	5
Peptic ulcer	44	48	92	5
Diabetes	63	22	85	4
Liver disease	17	60	77	4
Thyroid disease	31	42	73	4
Arteriosclerosis	69	2	71	4
Syphilis	4	54	58	
Gonorrhea	0	51	51	3
Stroke	6	39	45	2
Prostate gland trouble	11	30	41	2
Epilepsy	25	7	32	2
Cancer	11	12	23	1

[a]Illnesses are listed exactly as asked, except that the alternative wordings permitted to the interviewer (e.g., "arteriosclerosis, hardening of the arteries") are sometimes omitted.

[b]Excluding tuberculosis.

A-7. Present illnesses reported by adults at intake, by age group (in per cent).

Illnesses	(N=134) 18-20	(N=541) 21-30	(N=425) 31-40	(N=257) 41-50	(N=231) 51-59	(N=99) 60-64	(N=293) 65-up	(N=1,980) Total
Suffer from nerves	36	45	45	51	44	49	45	45
Arthritis	2	2	7	19	22	30	39	14
Varicose veins	6	10	10	12	22	14	24	14
Sinus trouble	17	11	11	16	15	12	15	13
Allergies	12	11	11	13	11	10	7	11
Heart trouble	3	4	6	9	15	24	23	10
Hypertension	3	5	6	11	15	20	22	10
Asthma	8	1	3	6	7	10	8	7
Severe anemia	5	5	4	5	5	6	7	5
Hemorrhoids	2	4	5	5	5	11	9	5
Kidney, bladder disease	2	3	2	4	5	5	7	5
Women's trouble	4	6	5	4	10	0	1	4
Diabetes	1	1	2	4	7	7	4	3
Arteriosclerosis	0	—[a]	1	2	3	7	16	3
Serious lung trouble	2	3	2	5	9	4	3	3
Hernia	0	—	3	2	5	8	8	3
Thyroid disease	1	1	—	5	2	4	1	2
Peptic ulcer	0	1	2	2	2	1	2	2
Cancer	0	—	—	2	1	2	1	2
Epilepsy	2	1	1	2	1	0	—	1
Gallstones	1	—	1	2	0	0	2	1
Liver disease	1	—	—	1	2	2	2	1
Parasites or worms	2	1	1	0	0	1	0	1
Prostate gland trouble	0	—	1	1	1	4	0	1
Rheumatic fever	2	1	1	1	3	3	1	1
Tuberculosis	1	—	1	1	1	2	1	1
Tumor	1	1	2	2	—	0	1	1
Stroke	0	—	0	0	—	0	1	1
Syphilis	0	—	0	—	0	0	0	—
Gonorrhea	0	0	0	0	0	0	0	0

[a]Dash signifies less than 1 per cent.

A-8. Doctor-patient agreement on the patient's illnesses in a sample of patients seen by Project doctors (255 patients).

	Person reporting the illness				
Illness	Doctor and patient	Patient only	Doctor only	Neither	Total
Suffer from nerves	130	10	27	88	255
Hypertension	33	24	17	181	255
Heart trouble	25	23	17	190	255
Arthritis	29	27	7	192	255
Varicose veins	35	18	7	195	255
Women's trouble	29	13	10	203	255
Lung trouble	25	10	14	206	255
Allergies	20	18	10	207	255
Hemorrhoids	24	22	2	207	255
Sinus trouble	18	26	1	210	255
Arteriosclerosis	8	9	26	212	255
Severe anemia	11	18	14	212	255
Tumor	24	9	10	212	255
Kidney, bladder	13	15	14	213	255
Hernia	18	10	1	226	255
Liver disease	7	8	12	228	255
Parasites	12	10	3	230	255
Asthma	17	4	3	231	255
Tuberculosis	11	7	5	232	255
Rheumatic fever	3	19	1	232	255
Gallstones	6	8	4	237	255
Syphilis	7	4	6	238	255
Thyroid disease	4	10	2	239	255
Prostate trouble	3	5	6	241	255
Gonorrhea	6	4	4	241	255
Ulcers	5	8	1	241	255
Cancer	4	2	7	242	255
Diabetes	7	3	3	242	255
Stroke	6	4	–	245	255
Epilepsy	4	2	3	245	255
Total	544	350	237	6,519	7,650

A-9. Symptoms reported by adults at intake (N=1,980).

Symptoms	Number of adults	Per cent of adults
Cavities in teeth	1,001	51
Very depressed and blue recently	876	44
Trouble with eyes	826	42
Tired all the time for no special reason	700	35
Trouble sleeping	634	32
Frequent severe headaches	606	31
Often have to go to bed when sick	595	30
Weight loss without dieting	584	30
Frequent backaches	536	27
Difficulty breathing	483	24
Trouble with teeth, excl. cavities	480	24
Appetite usually poor	438	22
Continually troubled with aches and pains	413	21
Bad cough for several weeks	409	21
Begun to be constipated recently	370	19
Ankles very often swollen	333	17
Suffer from indigestion	331	17
Pain in chest	320	16
Trouble with hearing	317	16
Skin trouble	264	13
Joints ever painfully swollen	252	13
Trouble with urination	179	9
Bloody bowel movements within year	144	7
Coughed up blood within year	135	7
Often vomit	134	7
Begun to have diarrhea recently	112	6
Any unusual lumps on the body	106	5
Passed blood when urinating	46	2

		Per cent of 1,224 women
Often lie down with periods	187	15
Consistent vaginal discharge or itching	167	14
Irregular periods or bleeding between	160	13

A-10. Symptoms reported by adults at intake, by age group (in per cent).

Symptoms[a]	(N=134) 18–20	(N=541) 21–30	(N=425) 31–40	(N=257) 41–50	(N=231) 51–59	(N=99) 60–65	(N=293) 65-up	(N=1,980) Total
Cavities in teeth	62	63	58	53	42	33	24	51
Depressed and blue	33	41	42	51	52	60	42	44
Trouble with eyes	28	30	50	58	58	57	53	42
Tired all the time	27	31	30	40	48	54	36	35
Trouble sleeping	15	25	29	39	42	47	38	32
Severe headache	31	35	34	35	28	26	18	31
Often ill in bed	26	27	27	36	40	39	26	30
Weight loss	29	31	25	26	32	45	30	30
Frequent backaches	13	23	28	32	33	34	28	27
Trouble breathing	19	21	22	25	34	31	27	24
Teeth, not cavities	11	19	21	31	35	33	28	24
Poor appetite	19	23	21	25	23	25	21	22
Aches and pains	17	14	16	30	30	32	24	21
Bad cough	21	19	19	24	26	24	18	21
Constipated lately	13	14	16	23	22	20	29	19
Indigestion	8	12	16	21	20	23	22	17
V. swollen ankles	8	10	13	20	28	28	24	17
Trouble hearing	8	8	8	19	23	20	36	16
Pain in chest	12	11	15	18	24	27	18	16
Skin trouble	13	13	10	14	17	20	14	13
Swollen joints	4	6	11	15	20	26	20	13
Trouble urinating	4	6	7	10	14	7	16	9
Bloody bowel movements	3	7	7	8	12	9	5	7
Coughed up blood	4	6	8	6	8	11	6	7
Often vomit	5	7	8	10	8	10	3	7
Diarrhea lately	5	5	5	8	4	13	5	6
Unusual lumps	5	4	4	4	5	4	9	5
Blood in urine	2	2	2	3	4	1	2	2

[a]For a full definition of each symptom-question abbreviated in this and later tables, see Table A-9 or the Health Questionnaire in Appendix B.

A-11. Distribution of responses about readiness to see a doctor for specific conditions, by general readiness to see a doctor (in per cent, N=1,643).

Conditions	See doctor right away	Wait awhile	Put off seeing doctor
Coughing up blood	98	97	95
Unusual lump on body	97	96	94
Shortness of breath	93	87	81
Pain in chest	93	83	78
Bad cough for several weeks	91	79	73
Tired all the time, no reason	83	70	64
Frequent headaches	77	63	60
Feeling very depressed and blue	63	44	41
Sore throat, running nose, for a couple of days	64	41	30
Diarrhea or constipation for a couple of days	53	41	34

A-12. Response of study group to Project invitation by address at intake and ethnic group (total study group persons).

Address at intake	Puerto Rican			Negro			Non–Puerto Rican white			Total persons		
	Total invited	Came to NYH Number	Per cent	Total invited	Came to NYH Number	Per cent	Total invited	Came to NYH Number	Per cent	Total invited	Came to NYH Number	Per cent
6th–13th Street	600	218	36	101	46	46	152	65	24	853	329	38
14th–29th Street	135	77	51[a]	15	6)		131	73	56	281	156	56
30th–56th Street	21	8		12	10)	52	77	54	70	110	72	65
57th–95th Street	48	26	54	15	6)		253	175	69	316	207	66
96th–106th Street	503	171	34	350	184	53	91	36	40	944	391	41
Total	1,307	500	39	493	252	51	704	403	57	2,504	1,155	46

[a]Base too small to percentage.

A-13. Family groupings of Project patients attending the New York Hospital, showing size of family from which they came and proportion of family coming to the project.

Family grouping at intake	Family groups	Adults in this group	Adults who came Number	Adults who came Per cent	Children in group	Children who came Number	Children who came Per cent	Persons in group	Persons who came Number	Persons who came Per cent
Husband and wife, no children	23	46	37	79a	X	X		46	37	79
Related adults	8	17	13		X	X		17	13	
One parent, 1 child	47	47	43		47	39		94	82	
One parent, 2–3 children	76	76	57		182	131		258	188	
One parent, 4–5 children	26	26	20	79	107	83	75	133	103	76
One parent, 6+ children	7	7	5		50	39		57	44	
One parent, children + adult child	1	2	2		3	2		5	4	
One parent, children + grandparent	3	6	2		9	6		15	8	
Both parent, 1 child	15	30	25		15	12		45	37	
Both parents, 2–3 children	31	62	43		74	51		136	94	
Both parents, 4–5 children	32	64	44	70	139	88	63	203	132	65
Both parents, 6+ children	13	26	18		96	56		122	74	
Both parents, children + adult child	3	9	2		9	8		18	10	
Both parents, children + grandparent	2	6	3		9	2		15	5	
Other	3	4	1	...b	9	2	...	13	3	...
Total family members	290	428	315	74	749	519	69	1,177	834	71
Single adults	321	321	321		X	X		321	321	
Total persons	611	749	636		749	519		1,498	1,155	

a Adults of this group who came as per cent of all adults in this group, i.e., 50 = 79 per cent of 63

b Too few to percentage

A-14. Number of Project patients[a] making various numbers of visits to the general medical and pediatric clinics in the first year.

	Adults		Children			
	General medicine		Pediatric isolation		General pediatrics	
Number of visits	Patients	Visits	Patients	Visits	Patients	Visits
1	114		80		98	
2	63		48		81	
3	60	829	28	349	74	878
4	51		11		49	
5	41		9		40	
6	38		4		15	
7	33		5		9	
8	35	1,117	2	141	6	229
9	22		4		2	
10	18		3		1	
11	15		—		1	
12	12		—		—	
13	88	575	—	15	—	11
14	3		—		—	
15	8		1		—	
16	4					
17	3					
18	3	267				
19	2					
20	3					
21	2					
22	1					
23	1	156				
25	1					
44	1					
Total	542	2,944[b]	195	505[c]	376	1,118

[a] 605 adults and 412 children came in the first year, but not all attended the general clinics.

[b] 2,717 of these visits were to Project doctors.

[c] 436 of these visits were to Project doctors.

A-15. Diagnoses of adult Project patients, by system (_N_=684).

Disorder	Diagnoses	Patients
Infective and parasitic	103	93
Tuberculosis	54	
Syphilis[a]	19	
Other	30	
Neoplasms	46	42
Malignant	24	
Benign or unspecified	22	
Allergic, endocrine, metabolic, and nutritional	229	184
Asthma	31	
Hay fever	6	
Other allergies	32	
Thyroid disorders	19	
Diabetes	30	
Obesity	87	
Malnutrition	15	
Other	9	
Blood and blood-forming organs	62	60
Anemia	52	
Other	10	
Mental, psychoneurotic, and personality disorders	486	369
Mental deficiency	40	
Organic brain damage	28	
Psychosis	73	
Psychophysiological reaction	55	
Other psychoneurosis	93	
Alcoholism	60	
Personality disorder: transient situational	54	
Personality disorder: chronic	83	
Nervous system and sense organs	419	274
Cerebro-vascular accident or residue	17	
Cerebral arteriosclerosis without CVA	15	
Epilepsy	13	
Migraine	12	

Nervous system and sense organs (continued)

Neuralgia or neuritis	11	
Cataracts	47	
Refractive errors	102	
Other eye disorders	90	
Impaired hearing	50	
Other ear disorders	19	
Other	43	
Circulatory system	**409**	**270**
Rheumatic Heart disease	12	
Arteriosclerotic heart disease[b]	106	
Hypertensive cardiovascular disease	54	
Essential hypertension	65	
Other heart disease	13	
Varicose veins	72	
Hemorrhoids	19	
Peripheral vascular disease	26	
Other circulatory	42	
Respiratory system	**254**	**182**
Acute upper respiratory infection	73	
Tonsilitis	21	
Sinusitis	10	
Bronchitis	49	
Bronchiectasis	5	
Pulmonary emphysema	44	
Pneumonia	19	
Other	35	
Digestive system, dental disorders	**281**	**270**
Digestive system, excluding dental	**238**	**164**
Hiatus hernia	12	
Other hernia	31	
Ulcer, stomach	7	
Ulcer, duodenum	19	
Functional gastro-intestinal disorders	28	
Cholecystitis and cholelithiasis	25	
Cirrhosis of liver	33	
Diverticulitis	13	
Other	62	

A-15 (Continued)

Genito-urinary system	244	169
Menstrual disorders	18	
Pelvic inflammatory disease	5	
Menopause	16	
Other female genital	65	
Benign prostatic hypertrophy	28	
Other male genital	20	
Pyelonephritis	19	
Nephritis and nephrosis	5	
Cystitis	14	
Other urinary tract infection	15	
Other urinary disorder	39	
Pregnancies	64	51
Skin and cellular tissue	131	113
Boils, abscesses	12	
Other	119	
Bones and organs of movement	180	142
Rheumatoid arthritis	12	
Osteoarthritis	74	
Osteoporosis	15	
Bursitis or synovitis	9	
Other	70	
Congenital malformations	16	14
Heart	5	
Other	11	
Injuries	63	55
Major	44	
Minor	19	
Miscellaneous	47	45
Headaches	11	
Backaches	21	
Other symptoms	15	
No diagnosis (healthy)	3	3

[a]Only syphilis requiring treatment was recorded.

[b]Eleven with angina, 19 with myocardial infarction, 11 with both.

A-16. Diagnoses of adult Project patients compared with the Baltimore population and the New York Hospital general medical clinic patients (rates per 1,000).

Disorder	Baltimore (N=8,439)	General Medical Clinic (N=719)	Project (N=684)
Infective and parasitic	_[a]	231	_[a]
Tuberculosis	9	24	79
Syphilis	50	179	28
Other	—	28	44
Neoplasms	73	81	68
Malignant	2	24	35
Benign or unspecified	72	57	32
Allergic, endocrine, metabolic, and nutritional	_[a]	399	337
Asthma	13 ⎫	57	46 ⎧
Allergies	8 ⎬		47 ⎨
Hay fever	24 ⎭		9 ⎩
Thyroid	34	43	28
Diabetes	37	146	44
Obesity	177	136	128
Other	_[a]	17	35
Blood	_[a]	26	91
Anemia	30	24	76
Other	_[a]	3	15
Mental, psychoneurotic, and personality disorders	148	214	715
Psychoses	6	8	143
Psychoneuroses	69	135	137
Psychophysiological reaction	50	29	81
Mental deficiency		4 ⎧	59 ⎧
Alcoholism	21 ⎨	14 ⎨	88 ⎨
Other behavior disorders		24 ⎩	201 ⎩
Respiratory system	_[a]	241	383
Bronchitis	_[a]	28	72
Bronchiectasis	_[a]	13	7
Pulmonary emphysema	_[a]	90	65
Sinusitis	12 ⎫	110 ⎧	15 ⎧
Other	_[a] ⎭		218 ⎩
Digestive system: dental disorders		25	413
Digestive system, excluding dental	_[a]	257	763
Hernia	46	60	63
Ulcer, stomach/duodenum	_[a]	26	38
Functional gastro-intestinal	_[a]	39	41
Cholecystitis, cholelithiasis	19	31	37
Cirrhosis	_[a]	24	49
Other, excluding dental	_[a]	31	110

A-16 (Continued)

Genito-urinary system	X	255	359
Prostate disease	29	77[b]	41
Cervicitis	31	–	7
Menopause		28	24
Other female genital	94[a]	88	122
Other male genital	–[a]	88	29
Kidney disease	4[a]	19	35
Other urinary	–[a]	43	100
Deliveries and complications of pregnancy	–[a]	8	94
Nervous system and sense organs	–[a]	202	616
Cataracts	–[a]	129	69
Refractive errors	–[a]		150
Other eye disorders	6		132
Impaired hearing	26	57	74
Other ear disorders			28
CVA or residue	4	15[b]	25
Cerebral arteriosclerosis without CVA	–[b]		22
Neuralgia and neuritis	–[a]	19	16
Migraine	10	10	18
Epilepsy		13	19
Other CNS	15	38	63
Circulatory system	386	711	601
Rheumatic fever	0.1	0	0
RHD	11	0	0
ASHD	31	199	156
HCDV	69	147	79
Other heart	16	8	19
Hypertension without heart	91	93	96[b]
Arteriosclerosis	18	57	–
Varicose veins	60	76	106
Hemorrhoids	74	33	28
Peripheral vascular	18	51	38
Other			62
Skin	–[a]	95	193
Bones	–[a]	313	265
Osteoarthritis	91	170[b]	109
Rheumatoid arthritis	5	–[b]	18[b]
Other arthritis	7	–[b]	–[b]
Osteoporosis	–[a]	28	22
Other	–[a]	115	116
Congenital malformations	–[a]	11	93
Injuries	–a	19	93
Symptoms only	56	64	69
Backaches	15		31
Headaches		64	16
Other	41		22

[a]Information not available.

[b]Included in "other" category in this system.

A-17. Reasons for hospitalization of adult patients at the New York Hospital by service (N=684).

Disorder	Medicine	Surgery	Obstetrics-Gynecology	Emergency	Total
Infective and parasitic					
Tuberculosis	2	2		1	4
Other				1	1
Neoplasms					
Malignant	5	5			10
Benign or unspecified		5			5
Allergic, endocrine, metabolic, and nutritional					
Diabetes	1			1	2
Dehydration and malnutrition	2			1	3
Blood	3				3
Mental, psychoneurotic, and personality disorders	2				2
Nervous system and sense organs					
Cataracts		20			20
Other eye conditions		12			12
Ear conditions		4			4
Other	4				4
Circulatory					
Myocardial infarct	10				10
ASHD, no mention of M.I.	9				9
Congestive heart failure	5				5
Acute rheumatic fever	1				1
Generalized arteriosclerosis	2				2
Other	3	2			5

A-17 (Continued)

Respiratory					
Pneumonia	7				7
Tonsillitis	2	7			7
Other		5			7
Digestive					
Dental	1	10			10
Gallbladder	7	6			7
Liver	1				7
Ulcer		4			5
Hernia		5			5
Other	2	8		3	13
Genito-urinary					
Female genital			16		16
Prostate		4			4
Other male genital		2			2
Kidney	4	4		1	9
Other urinary		4			4
Delivery and complications of pregnancy					
Delivery			45		45
D & C			7		7
Antepartum complications			2		2
Skin					
Plastic Surgery	1	6	1		6
Abscess or cellulitis		2		2	6
Bone and organs of movement					
Muscular dystrophy	1	1			1

					Total
Congenital malformations					
Congenital heart disease	1				1
Cleft palate		1			1
Injuries					
Burn				1	1
Fracture		8			8
Head injury		1			1
Miscellaneous					
Abdominal pain	2	2			4
Poisoning	1			1	2
Fever of unknown origin				1	1
Total	79	132	71	12	294

A-18. Significant factors interfering with effective care of adult patients (N=684).

Patient factors	Number of patients with each factor	Per cent of patients with any of these
Factor		
Patient did not come in, whereabouts unknown	180	
Patient did not come in, whereabouts known	30	
Language	21	30
Socio-cultural	32	
Intellectual	37	
Administrative defects		
Patients' appointment not sent	20	
Reports not available	5	
Referral appointment not made	10	
Social Service referrals not made	4	
Tests not arranged	4	
Chart not obtained when requested, undesirable consequences	13	19
Inability to coordinate with NYH in-patient	5	
Inability to coordinate with NYH other clinics	6	
Inability to coordinate with other institutions	6	
Patient geographically inaccessible	14	
Other administrative defects	21	
Professional defects		
Inadequate history	6	
Inadequate physical exam	6	
Inadequate laboratory	5	
Inadequate social-psychological data	19	
Inadequate formulation of problem	9	
Inadequate treatment	5	
Inadequate follow-up	23	15
Psychiatric evaluation inadequate	36	
Psychiatric follow-up inadequate	24	
Social Service evaluation incomplete	7	
Social Service follow-up incomplete	18	
Social Service referral needed, not made	3	
Facilities unavailable		
Sheltered workshops	37	
Housing for elderly or handicapped	23	
Public housing	12	
Vocational training for handicapped	8	13
Day nurseries	3	
Other	15	
No factors interfering with care	280	41

A-19. Diagnoses of pediatric Project patients who had serious medical problems at intake, by medical care status at that time.

Disorder	No care (25 children)	Inadequate care (25 children)	Adequate care (16 children)	Total (66 children)
Primary tuberculosis	6[a]	–	–	6
Exposure to tuberculosis	2	4	–	6
Asthma	2[b]	2	1	5
Malnutrition	–	2	1	3
Obesity	–	1	–	1
Anemia	4[c]	4[d]	–	8
Psychiatric disorders	3	4	–	7
Mental retardation	1	4[e]	–	5
Organic brain syndrome	–	–	1	2
Seizure disorder	1	–	–	1
Hearing loss	3	1	–	4
Deaf-mutism	–	–	3[f]	3
Rheumatic heart disease	–	1	1	2
Hernia, inguinal	2	–	–	2
Chronic nephritis	–	–	1	1
Severe atopic dermatitis	–	–	1	1
Port wine stain, face	1	–	–	1
Congenital heart disease	–	–	3[g]	3
Genito-urinary tract anomaly	1	–	–	1
Anomalies of face and ear	1	–	–	1
Prematurity	–	–	3	3
Severe scars, secondary to third degree burns	–	1	–	1
Other	1	3	1	5

[a]Four were members of the same family. 1 is the child with congenital anomalies of face and ear.

[b]These are the same children as the 2 exposed to tuberculosis.

[c]One was secondary to severe menometrorrhagia, which was untreated.

[d]Two were siblings with sickle cell anemia, the other 2 are the 2 with malnutrition.

[e]One had cerebral palsy as well.

[f]Two were members of the same family.

[g]One had Down's syndrome as well.

A-20. Diagnoses of pediatric Project patients, by system (*N*=520).

Disorder	Diagnoses	Patients
Infective and parasitic	150	124
Tuberculosis–primary active	9	
Tuberculosis–primary inactive	10	
Active contagion	57	
Other infective	26	
Parasitic	48	
Neoplasms, benign or unspecified	3	3
Allergic, endocrine, metabolic, and nutritional	90	73
Asthma	26	
Other allergies	29	
Obesity	17	
Malnutrition	10	
Other endocrine or nutritional	8	
Blood and blood-forming organs	118	106
Anemia	66	
Other	52	
Mental, psychoneurotic, and personality disorders	147	100
Mental deficiency	27	
Organic brain damage	2	
Psychosis	2	
Psychoneurosis, including psychophysiological reaction	7	
Personality disorder–transient situational	9	
Personality disorder–chronic	3	
Behavior disorders	34	
School adjustment problems	42	
Enuresis	21	
Nervous system and sense organs	116	105
Convulsive disorders	9	
Refractive errors	45	
Other eye disorders	40	
Impaired hearing	7	
Other ear disorders	5	
Other	10	
Respiratory system	578	309
Acute upper respiratory infection	181	
Sinusitis, bronchitis, bronchiolitis, otitis	160	

Respiratory system (continued)

Tonsillitis, pharyngitis	173	
Pneumonia	18	
Other	46	
Digestive system: dental	106	102
Dental caries	98	
Other dental	8	
Digestive system, excluding dental	93	69
Gastro-enteritis	50	
Functional gastro-intestinal disorders	8	
Hernia: inguinal	5	
Hernia: umbilical	8	
Other	22	
Genito-urinary system	37	33
Menstrual disorders	2	
Other female genital	1	
Phimosis	16	
Other male genital	6	
Nephritis and nephrosis	3	
Urinary tract infection	4	
Other urinary	5	
Skin and cellular tissue	145	117
Boils, abscesses	11	
Other	134	
Bones and organs of movement	30	28
Congenital malformations	17	16
Heart	4	
Other	13	
Injuries	87	75
Major	12	
Minor	75	
Miscellaneous	105	99
Prematurity	6	
History of prematurity	7	
Headache	9	
Other symptoms	20	
Small stature	54	
Other diagnoses	9	
No diagnoses (healthy)	28	28

A-21. Selected psychiatric diagnoses, comparing children and adults seen on the Project.

Disorder	Children (N=520)		Adults (N=684)	
	Number	Per cent	Number	Per cent
Mental deficiency	27	5.2	40	5.8
Psychoneurosis	4	0.8	93	13.6
Chronic personality disorder	3	.6	83	12.1
Psychosis	2	.4	73	10.7
Alcoholism	—	—	60	8.8

A-22. Reasons for hospitalization of pediatric Project patients at the New York Hospital (*N*=520).

Disorder	Admission
Tuberculosis	1
Benign neoplasm	1
Anemia	2
Eye disorders	2
Intracranial hemmorhage	1
Rheumatic fever	2
Pneumonia	5
Tonsillitis	17
Bronchiolitis	1
Other respiratory	1
Dental	2
Hernia	3
Appendicitis	1
Gastroenteritis	2
Circumcision	5
Kidney disease	3
Trabeculated bladder	1
Skin graft	3
Abscess	1
Cellulitis	2
Congenital heart disease	3
Other congenital anomalies	2
Prematurity	3
Poisoning	5
Miscellaneous	2
Total	73

A-23. Significant factors interfering with effective care of pediatric patients (*N*=520).

Factor	Number of patients with each factor	Per cent of patients with any of these
Patient factors		
Patient did not come in, whereabouts known	172	
Patient did not come in, whereabouts unknown	23	43
Language barrier	36	
Socio-cultural barrier	43	
Intellectual barrier	23	
Administrative defects		
Patients' appointment not sent	9	
Reports not available	4	
Referral appointments not made (including Social Service)	4	
Tests not arranged	1	
Inability to coordinate with NYH in-patient	2	
Inability to coordinate with NYH other clinics	6	13
Inability to coordinate with other institutions	8	
Patient geographically inaccessible	18	
Other administrative defects	25	
Professional defects		
Inadequate history	15	
Inadequate physical exam	5	
Inadequate laboratory	23	
Inadequate socio-psychological data	9	
Inadequate formulation of problem	1	
Inadequate treatment	4	10
Inadequate follow-up	10	
Psychiatric evaluation inadequate	1	
Social Service evaluation incomplete	4	
Social Service follow-up incomplete	2	
Social Service referrals needed, not made	1	
Facilities unavailable	2	—[a]
No factors interfering with care	235	45

[a]Less than 1 per cent.

A-24. Summary on use of New York Hospital out-patient services by study group, first year.

Group	Persons at risk	Persons coming that year Number	Per cent	Total visits	Visits per person coming that year	Visits per person at risk
A						
Aged	99	72	73	755	10.8	7.6
Disabled	118	88	75	1,032	11.7	8.7
Unemployed	60	41	68	478	11.6	7.8
Total Single	277	201	73	2,265	11.3	8.2
Family adults	342	156	96	1,123	7.2	3.3
Teenagers	101	32	32	131	4.1	1.3
Children	611	296	48	1,561	5.3	2.6
Total Family	1,054	484	46	2,815	5.8	2.7
Total	1,331	685	51	5,078	7.4	3.8
B						
Aged	71	44	62	467	10.6	6.6
Disabled	92	64	70	697	11.2	7.5
Unemployed	93	43	46	412	9.6	6.4
Total Single	256	151	59	1,576	10.6	6.2
Family adults	322	71	22	417	5.8	1.3
Teenagers	76	19	25	83	4.4	1.1
Children	519	104	20	535	5.1	1.0
Total Family	917	194	21	1,035	5.3	1.1
Total	1,173	345	29	2,611	7.6	2.2
A+B						
Aged	170	116	68	1,222	10.5	7.2
Disabled	210	152	72	1,729	11.5	8.2
Unemployed	153	84	55	890	10.6	5.8
Total Single	533	352	66	3,841	11.0	7.2
Family adults	664	227	34	1,540	6.8	2.3
Teenagers	177	51	29	214	4.1	1.2
Children	1,130	400	35	2,096	5.2	1.9
Total Family	1,971	678	34	3,850	5.7	2.0
Total	2,504	1,030	41	7,689	7.5	3.1

A-25. Summary on use of New York Hospital out-patient services by study group, second year.

Group	Persons at risk	Persons coming that year Number	Per cent	Total visits	Visits per person coming that year	Visits per person at risk
A						
Aged	91	59	65	568	9.6	6.2
Disabled	111	62	56	678	10.9	6.1
Unemployed	59	27	46	233	8.6	3.9
Total Single	261	148	57	1,479	10.0	5.7
Family adults	342	121	35	810	6.7	2.4
Teenagers	101	30	30	132	4.4	1.3
Children	610	258	42	1,274	4.9	2.1
Total Family	1,053	409	39	2,216	5.4	2.1
Total	1,315	557	42	3,695	6.6	2.8
B						
Aged	68	35	51	376	10.7	5.5
Disabled	83	38	46	403	10.6	4.9
Unemployed	93	38	41	340	8.9	3.7
Total Single	244	111	45	1,119	10.1	4.6
Family adults	320	60	19	450	7.5	1.4
Teenagers	76	14	18	56	4.0	0.7
Children	518	102	20	519	5.1	1.0
Total Family	914	176	19	1,025	5.8	1.1
Total	1,158	287	25	2,144	7.5	1.9
A+B						
Aged	159	94	59	944	10.0	5.9
Disabled	194	100	52	1,081	10.8	5.6
Unemployed	152	65	43	573	8.8	3.8
Total Single	505	259	51	2,598	10.0	5.1
Family adults	662	181	27	1,261	7.0	1.9
Teenagers	177	44	25	188	4.3	1.1
Children	1,128	360	32	1,826	5.1	1.6
Total Family	1,967	585	30	3,275	5.6	1.7
Total	2,473	844	34	5,839	6.9	2.4

A-26. Distribution of costs of in-patient care incurred by study group at the New York Hospital (in dollars).

Category	First year	Second year
Surgical procedures	11,703	6,696
Laboratory tests and X rays	12,364	9,137
Bed cost	82,744	57,580
Total	106,811	73,413

A-27. Summary on utilization of New York Hospital in-patient services by study group, first year.

Group	Persons coming that year	Persons admitted Number	Per cent	Admissions	Days	Average length of stay
A						
Aged	72	22	31	28	460	16.4
Disabled	88	18	20	21	345	16.4
Unemployed	41	9	22	11	143	13.0
Total Single	201	49	24	60	948	15.8
Family adults	156	34	22	38	309	8.1
Teenagers	32	3	9	3	8	2.7
Children	296	23	8	27	113	4.2
Total Family	484	60	12	68	430	6.3
Total	685	109	16	128	1,378	10.8
B						
Aged	44	13	30	17	273	16.1
Disabled	64	11	17	17	207	12.2
Unemployed	43	16	37	21	275	13.1
Total Single	151	40	26	55	755	13.7
Family adults	71	19	27	26	252	10.0
Teenagers	19	1	5	2	7	3.5
Children	104	9	9	10	88	11.5
Total Family	194	29	15	38	347	9.1
Total	345	69	20	93	1,102	11.8
A+B						
Aged	116	35	30	45	733	16.3
Disabled	152	29	19	38	552	14.5
Unemployed	84	25	30	32	418	13.1
Total Single	352	89	25	115	1,703	14.8
Family adults	227	53	23	64	561	8.8
Teenagers	51	4	8	5	15	3.0
Children	400	32	8	37	201	5.4
Total Family	678	89	13	106	777	7.3
Total	1,030	178	17	221	2,480	11.2

A-28. Summary on utilization of New York Hospital in-patient services by study group, second year.

Group	Persons coming that year	Persons admitted Number	Per cent	Admissions	Days	Average length of stay
A						
Aged	59	16	27	20	325	16.2
Disabled	62	13	21	14	150	10.7
Unemployed	27	3	11	3	13	4.3
Total Single	148	32	20	37	488	13.2
Family adults	121	23	22	28	250	8.9
Teenagers	30	2	7	2	11	5.5
Children	258	13	5	16	126	7.9
Total Family	409	38	9	46	387	8.4
Total	557	70	13	83	875	10.5
B						
Aged	35	11	31	13	307	23.6
Disabled	38	6	16	7	181	25.9
Unemployed	38	8	21	8	146	18.3
Total Single	111	25	23	28	634	22.6
Family adults	60	10	17	12	152	12.7
Teenagers	14	2	14	3	13	4.3
Children	102	7	7	7	51	7.3
Total Family	176	19	11	22	216	9.8
Total	287	44	15	50	850	17.0
A+B						
Aged	94	27	29	33	632	19.2
Disabled	100	19	19	21	331	15.8
Unemployed	65	11	17	11	159	14.5
Total Single	259	57	22	65	1,122	17.3
Family adults	181	33	18	40	402	10.0
Teenagers	44	4	9	5	24	4.8
Children	360	20	6	23	177	7.7
Total Family	585	57	10	68	603	8.9
Total	844	114	14	133	1,725	13.0

A-29. Summary on costs of New York Hospital in-patient services incurred by study group, first year (in dollars).

Group	Total cost	Cost per person at risk	Cost per person coming that year	Cost per admission
A				
Aged	18,181	184	253	649
Disabled	13,709	116	156	652
Unemployed	5,510	92	134	501
Total Single	37,400	135	186	623
Family adults	14,392	42	92	379
Teenagers	427	4	13	143
Children	5,608	7	19	208
Total Family	20,428	19	42	300
Total	57,828	43	84	452
B				
Aged	12,939	182	294	762
Disabled	9,432	103	152	555
Unemployed	11,033	119	257	525
Total Single	33,404	130	224	607
Family adults	11,202	35	156	631
Teenagers	312	4	16	156
Children	4,063	8	39	406
Total Family	15,577	17	80	410
Total	48,981	42	162	527
A+B				
Aged	31,120	183	269	692
Disabled	23,141	110	154	609
Unemployed	16,543	108	197	517
Total Single	70,804	133	202	616
Family adults	25,594	39	112	400
Teenagers	739	4	14	148
Children	9,674	9	24	261
Total Family	36,007	18	53	340
Total	106,811	43	104	483

A-30. Summary on cost of New York Hospital in-patient services incurred by study group, second year (in dollars).

Group	Total cost	Cost per person at risk	Cost per person coming that year	Cost per admission
A				
Aged	12,744	140	216	637
Disabled	6,322	57	102	452
Unemployed	667	11	25	222
Total Single	19,733	76	133	533
Family adults	11,416	33	94	408
Teenagers	434	4	14	217
Children	7,060	12	27	292
Total Family	18,910	18	46	394
Total	38,644	29	69	455
B				
Aged	10,890	160	311	838
Disabled	8,221	99	216	1,174
Unemployed	6,615	69	169	801
Total Single	25,526	105	230	912
Family adults	6,742	21	112	562
Teenagers	673	9	48	224
Children	1,827	4	18	365
Total Family	9,243	10	52	462
Total	34,769	30	121	740
A+B				
Aged	23,635	149	251	716
Disabled	14,543	75	145	693
Unemployed	7,081	47	109	644
Total Single	45,259	90	175	696
Family adults	18,159	27	100	454
Teenagers	1,108	6	25	222
Children	8,888	8	25	384
Total Family	28,154	14	48	414
Total	73,413	30	87	552

A-31. Per person cost of New York Hospital in-patient care by year and age.

Age at intake	Persons at risk	Persons who came that year		Cost per person at risk	Cost per person who came that year
		Number	Per cent		
First year					
Under 13	1,130	400	35	$ 8.56	$ 24.18
13–17	179	51	28	4.12	14.49
18–29	359	119	34	32.11	96.90
30–49	443	202	46	48.12	105.55
50–64	219	137	63	147.34	235.54
65 or over	174	121	70	179.75	258.49
Total	2,504	1,030	41	$ 42.66	$103.70
Second year					
Under 13	1,128	359	32	7.88	24.76
13–17	179	444	25	6.18	25.16
18–29	358	77	22	17.93	83.61
30–49	435	153	35	32.12	93.01
50–64	209	111	53	87.41	172.47
65 or over	164	100	62	135.82	236.34
Total	2,473	844	34	$ 29.70	$ 82.02

A-32. Per admission cost of New York Hospital in-patient care by year and sex.

Sex	Persons at risk	Persons who came that year		Persons admitted	Admissions	Cost per admission
		Number	Per cent			
First year						
Male	1,108	446	40	70	95	$572
Female	1,396	584	42	108	126	385
Second year						
Male	1,090	360	33	53	69	$630
Female	1,383	484	35	61	64	441

A-33. Citywide comparison of study and control group: percentage of ambulant care rendered by the various sources, by group and year (in per cent).

Source of care	First year A (N=1,331)	First year B (N=1,173)	First year C (N=1,685)	Second year A (N=1,315)	Second year B (N=1,158)	Second year C (N=1,667)
Hospital out-patient department and emergency room						
New York Hospital	53.2	33.8	4.0	58.7	35.1	4.4
Mt. Sinai	5.9	6.8	10.7	3.6	7.6	10.9
Other voluntary	5.9	6.7	8.4	2.5	5.5	12.2
Bellevue	10.5	17.6	27.4	10.8	19.8	25.3
Metropolitan	6.5	12.4	17.4	6.3	9.0	14.6
Other city	1.1	2.0	1.2	0.5	4.2	2.4
Total	83.1	79.3	69.1	82.7	81.4	69.8
Non-hospital clinics						
Child health stations	1.7	5.4	5.3	1.8	2.7	4.0
Dental clinics	9.6	10.1	14.4	7.4	9.8	12.4
Other clinics	2.1	1.8	2.7	4.2	1.6	2.0
Total	13.4	17.3	22.4	13.2	14.1	18.4
Doctors						
Private	2.6	2.8	4.6	3.8	4.0	7.6
Welfare	0.9	0.6	3.9	0.3	0.4	4.2
Total	3.5	3.4	8.5	4.1	4.4	11.9
Total	100.0	100.0	100.0	100.0	100.0	100.0

A-34. Citywide admissions to general hospitals by group and year showing minimum (recorded) and probable (adjusted) figures (rates per 1,000 persons).

Group	Admissions	Days	Average stay
First year			
A (appointment)	181–201	2,308–2,610	12.8–13.0
B (demand)	181–210	2,388–2,838	13.2–13.5
C (control)	136–170	1,878–2,467	13.8–14.5
Second year			
A (appointment)	129–149	1,524–1,799	11.8–12.1
B (demand)	122–151	2,002–2,532	16.4–16.8
C (control)	81–102	1,138–1,510	14.0–14.8

A-35. Citywide admissions for childbirth by group and year (rates per 1,000).

Group	Admissions	Days	Average stay
First year			
A (appointment)	41	224	5.4
B (demand)	38	192	5.1
C (control)	40	218	5.5
Second year			
A (appointment)	25	134	5.4
B (demand)	20	144	7.2[a]
C (control	22	92	4.2

[a]This rate is raised by one long admission involving postpartum complications. If this admission is excluded, the average stay is 4.7.

A-36. Citywide admissions to general hospitals (deliveries excluded) by group and year (rates per 1,000).

Group	Admissions	Days	Average stay
First year			
A (appointment)	140–160	2,084–2,386	14.9
B (demand)	143–172	2,196–2,646	15.3
C (control)	96–130	1,660–2,249	17.4
Second year			
A (appointment)	104–124	1,390–1,665	13.4
B (demand)	102–131	1,858–2,388	18.2
C (control)	59–80	1,046–1,418	17.6

A-37. Citywide long-term general hospitalizations 30 days or over by group and year (rates per 1,000)[a].

Group	Admissions	Days	Average stay
First year			
A	13	672	52.6
B	17	915	53.6
C	9	594	65.4
Second year			
A	11	652	57.2
B	19	1,100	57.9
C	6	307	51.1

[a]Because it is believed unlikely that many of these would have been missed, a correction factor has not been added in this table. These are recorded hospitalizations.

A-38. Persons in long-term institutions, by group and year (rates per 1,000).

Group	State mental hospital	Chronic hospital	Nursing home	Home care	Any of these institutions
First year only					
A study group	2	2	3	1	8[a]
B study group	2	1	1	2	4[b]
C control group	1	1	4	1	5[c]
Both years					
A	8	2	8	4	22
B	8	3	8	1	20
C	5	1	4	2	11
Second year only					
A	7	5	4	2	15
B	5	4	3	2	14
C	4	5	1	1	10
Total					
A	17	9	15	7	45
B	15	8	12	5	38
C	10	7	9	4	26

[a] 3 died.

[b] 1 died.

[c] 3 died.

A-39. Citywide comparison of study and control groups: calculated cost of ambulant care per person at risk, by source of care (in dollars).

	Study group		
Source of care	A	B	Control group (C)
First year			
New York Hospital clinics	46.4	25.7	2.8
Other voluntary hospital clinics	9.7	9.7	12.7
City hospital clinics	10.0	15.5	20.2
Non-hospital clinics	7.1	7.4	9.1
Non-clinic care	1.5	1.3	2.8
Total	74.7	59.6	47.6
Second year			
New York Hospital	43.3	19.8	2.2
Other voluntary hospital clinics	4.1	5.5	10.5
City hospital clinics	6.7	12.0	13.0
Non-hospital clinics	2.5	1.8	1.7
Non-clinic care	1.3	1.2	2.8
Total	57.9	40.3	30.2

A-40. Results of record search in four main hospitals for study and control group births first year.

Result	New York Hospital	Bellevue	Metropolitan	Mount Sinai	Total
Mother's and child's chart found and abstracted	28	19	30	12	89
One but not both charts found and abstracted	1	29	1	0	31
Mother's name in index, chart not available	0	6	2	0	8
Mother's name not in index	1	5	2	1	9
Total reported	30	59	35	13	137

A-41. Respondents' attitude toward Bellevue, before and after Project, by response group.

	Study Group											
	Came and stayed				Came and went				Didn't come			
	Before		After		Before		After		Before		After	
Items endorsed	Number	Per cent	Number	Per cent	Number	Per cent	Number	Per cent	Number	Per cent	Number	Per cent
Easy to get to	150	19	100	16	46	24	37	24	153	22	107	20
Good, but too far away	34	4	22	4	4	2	3	2	21	3	20	4
Only for rich people	1	...[a]	4	1	0	0	0	0	2	...	0	0
Has the best doctors	108	14	56	9	30	15	32	21	104	15	97	19
Friendly	83	11	19	3	27	14	13	9	81	12	60	12
Keeps you waiting much too long	109	14	91	15	23	12	16	11	104	15	73	14
Overcrowded	137	17	145	23	31	16	27	18	121	18	81	16
Not enough doctors and nurses	51	7	49	8	14	7	10	6	36	5	25	5
Gloomy, or dirty	76	10	83	14	10	5	10	6	35	5	39	7
Doesn't treat you like a person	32	4	44	7	10	5	5	3	32	5	16	3
Total responses	781	100	613	100	195	100	153	100	689	100	518	100
Persons interviewed[b]	404		375		99		95		313		242	

[a]Less than 1 per cent.

[b]Table omits the study group respondents (191 before, 25 after) who could not be classified for intentions to stay.

(Continued)

A-41 (Continued)

| Items endorsed | Control Group | | | |
| | Before | | After | |
	Number	Per cent	Number	Per cent
Easy to get to	283	22	154	17
Good, but too far away	44	3	63	7
Only for rich people	0	0	3	...
Has the best doctors	227	18	184	20
Friendly	158	13	89	10
Keeps you waiting much too long	174	14	128	14
Overcrowded	196	16	157	18
Not enough doctors and nurses	60	5	29	3
Gloomy, or dirty	74	6	68	8
Doesn't treat you like a person	42	3	29	3
Total responses	1,258	100	904	100
Persons interviewed [b]	636		463	

A-42. Attitude toward Metropolitan, before and after Project, by response group.

	Study Group											
	Came and Stayed				Came and Went				Didn't Come			
	Before		After		Before		After		Before		After	
Items endorsed	Number	Per cent	Number	Per cent	Number	Per cent	Number	Per cent	Number	Per cent	Number	Per cent
Easy to get to	113	24	76	18	27	24	18	18	87	23	65	23
Good, but too far away	13	3	3	1	4	4	3	3	9	3	4	1
Only for rich people	2	...[a]	0	0	0	0	0	0	3	1	0	0
Has the best doctors	23	5	6	1	8	7	6	6	15	4	13	4
Friendly	56	12	18	4	16	14	11	11	36	9	35	13
Keeps you waiting much too long	77	16	85	20	21	19	19	19	57	19	52	18
Overcrowded	87	18	93	21	20	18	20	20	84	23	58	20
Not enough doctors and nurses	44	9	66	15	6	6	9	9	34	9	25	9
Gloomy, or dirty	28	6	45	10	4	4	7	7	20	5	15	5
Doesn't treat you like a person	34	7	42	10	4	4	7	7	29	8	23	8
Total responses	477	100	434	100	110	100	100	100	374	100	290	100
Persons interviewed	404		375		99		95		313		242	

[a]Less than 1 per cent.

A-42 (Continued)

	Control Group			
	Before		After	
Items endorsed	Number	Per cent	Number	Per cent
Easy to get to	160	21	104	18
Good, but too far away	30	4	20	4
Only for rich people	3	...	2	...
Has the best doctors	38	5	26	5
Friendly	95	12	67	12
Keeps you waiting much too long	126	17	92	16
Overcrowded	149	20	123	22
Not enough doctors and nurses	69	9	61	11
Gloomy, or dirty	31	4	27	5
Doesn't treat you like a person	56	8	41	7
Total responses	757	100	573	100
Persons interviewed	636		463	

A-43. Attitude toward Mount Sinai, before and after Project, by response group.

	Study Group											
	Came and Stayed				Came and Went				Didn't Come			
	Before		After		Before		After		Before		After	
Items endorsed	Number	Per cent	Number	Per cent	Number	Per cent	Number	Per cent	Number	Per cent	Number	Per cent
Easy to get to	46	20	42	25	13	21	14	23	44	18	38	20
Good, but too far away	30	13	16	9	5	7	5	7	19	8	8	4
Only for rich people	36	15	28	16	7	11	7	11	37	15	22	12
Has the best doctors	37	16	23	14	13	21	6	10	53	21	33	17
Friendly	30	13	15	9	12	19	14	23	40	16	34	18
Keeps you waiting much too long	26	11	27	16	7	11	7	11	25	10	28	15
Overcrowded	15	6	11	6	3	5	5	7	17	7	18	9
Not enough doctors and nurses	9	4	6	4	3	5	4	6	8	3	5	3
Gloomy, or dirty	1	—a	0	0	1	2	0	0	1	1	1	1
Doesn't treat you like a person	4	2	2	1	0	0	0	0	4	2	2	1
Total responses	234	100	170	100	63	100	63	100	247	100	189	100
Persons interviewed	404		375		99		95		313		242	

a Less than 1 per cent.

A-43 (Continued)

Items endorsed	Control Group			
	Before		After	
	Number	Per cent	Number	Per cent
Easy to get to	95	22	64	18
Good, but too far away	50	11	43	12
Only for rich people	44	10	34	10
Has the best doctors	83	19	68	20
Friendly	87	20	67	19
Keeps you waiting much too long	30	7	28	8
Overcrowded	37	8	29	8
Not enough doctors and nurses	6	1	10	3
Gloomy, or dirty	2	1	1	—
Doesn't treat you like a person	4	1	6	2
Total responses	438	100	350	100
Persons interviewed	636		463	

Appendix B
Questionnaires

NATIONAL OPINION
RESEARCH CENTER
Univ. of Chicago

CONFIDENTIAL
Survey 438
7-61

Health Care Study

Attitude Questionnaire

---

1. A. Would you say your own health, in general, is excellent, good, fair, or poor?

   B. IF SPOUSE IN CASE: How about the health of your (spouse) – In general, would you rate it as excellent, good, fair, or poor?

   C. IF CHILDREN UNDER 18 IN CASE: How about the health of the child(ren), in general?

	A. Self	B. Spouse	C. Children
Excellent	6-1*	7-1	8-1
Good	2*	2	2
Fair	3**	3	3
Poor	4**	4	4
Don't know	5**	5	5

   *D. IF OWN HEALTH "EXCELLENT" OR "GOOD": Are there any small things that bother you? (What?)

   9-

   10-

   **E. IF OWN HEALTH "FAIR", "POOR" OR "DON'T KNOW": What are the main things that bother you? (Anything else?)

   11-

   12-

---

2. A. Would you say you think about your health fairly often, once in a while, or hardly ever?

   B. Do you talk about your health with your family and friends fairly often, once in a while, or hardly ever?

	A Think About	B Talk About
Fairly often	13-1	14-1
Once in a while	2	2
Hardly ever	3	3
Don't know	4	4

3. During the last twelve months, have you seen a doctor for any reason about your own health?

Yes	15-1*
No	2

*A. IF "YES": Have you been entirely satisfied with the care and treatment you got from doctors during the last twelve months, or were there some things about the care that you were not satisfied with?

Entirely satisfied	16-1
Some things not	2**
Don't know	3

**B. IF "SOME THINGS NOT": What was that?

17-

18-

---

4. A. If you had to go to the hospital as a bed patient, which hospital in New York City would you choose, if you could go wherever you liked?

19-

20-

B. Why that one?

21-

22-

C. Is there anything (else) you especially like about that hospital?

23-

---

5. A. And which hospital in New York City would you *least* like to go to?

24-

25-

B. Why that one?

26-

27-

C. Is there anything (else) you don't like about that hospital?

28-

6. A. If you had to go to a *clinic* for medical care, which clinic would you choose in New York City, if you could go wherever you liked?

29-

30-

B. IF DIFFERENT FROM HOSPITAL NAMED IN Q.4: Why that one?

31-

32-

---

7. If you could choose, and it didn't cost you anything, would you rather go to a *hospital* clinic or emergency room, or would you rather see a private doctor?

Clinic or emergency room	33-1*
Private doctor	2*
Don't know	3

*A. IF "CLINIC OR EMERGENCY ROOM" OR "PRIVATE DOCTOR": Why?

34-

35-

---

8. When you go to a clinic, how important is it that you see the same doctor each time – is that very important to you, fairly important, or not important at all?

Very important	36-1
Fairly important	2
Not important	3
Don't know	4

---

9. Now I have some questions about doctors. Here are some words which describe different kinds of doctors. (*HAND RESPONDENT CORRECT SIDE OF CARD*)

Would you pick out three or four which describe the kind of doctor *you yourself* like best?

A. Young	37-1
B. Old	2
C. Man	3
D. Woman	4
E. Takes a personal interest	5
F. Doesn't ask unnecessary questions	6
G. Extra thorough and complete	7
H. Tries not to give me too much medicine	8
I. Tells me all I want to know about my illness	9
J. Speaks my own language	38-1
K. Is my own religion	2
L. Puts me at ease	3
M. Spends a lot of time with me	4
Don't know	5

10. Here are some things people sometimes say about doctors. I'd like to know whether you personally think they are true of *most* doctors, or not. For example (*Read "A"*). Do you think that's true of most doctors, or not? (*Continue through list, circling one code for each.*)

	True of most	Not True	Don't Know
A. They don't give you a chance to tell them exactly what your trouble is	39-1	2	3
B. They don't take enough personal interest in you	40-1	2	3
C. Doctors want you to come back for additional visits even if you don't need to	41-1	2	3
D. They don't tell you enough about your condition; they don't explain just what the trouble is	42-1	2	3
E. Doctors give better care to their private patients than to their clinic patients	43-1	2	3
F. They tell you there's nothing wrong with you when you know there is	44-1	2	3
G. Doctors hurt you when they examine you and make you feel worse than when you came in	45-1	2	3
H. Doctors rush too much when they examine you	46-1	2	3

---

11. A. If you had a chance to talk to a doctor for half an hour, at no cost to you, are there any things about your own health that you'd like to ask him?

Yes	47-1*
No	2
Don't know	3

*B. IF "YES": What sort of things would you ask him about? (Anything else?)

48-

49-

---

12. A. ASK ONLY IF SPOUSE OR CHILDREN UNDER 18 IN CASE: Are there any particular things you'd like to ask a doctor about the health of other members of your family?

Yes	50-1*
No	2
Don't know	3

*B. IF "YES": What sort of things? (Anything else?)

51-

52-

13. If you suddenly needed a doctor at night or on a Sunday, what would you do? (*Do NOT read answer categories.*)

Phone doctor	53-1
Send someone to get doctor	2
Call police or ambulance	3
Go to emergency room	4
Other (*specify*)	5
Don't know	6

14. How much trouble do you think you would have getting a doctor to come to your home at night or on a Sunday – a great deal of trouble, some trouble, or no trouble at all?

Great deal	54-1*
Some	2*
No trouble at all	3
Don't know	4

*A. IF "GREAT DEAL" OR "SOME": Would this bother you a great deal, or some, or not at all?

Great deal	55-1
Some	2
Not at all	3
Don't know	4

15. Suppose you went to the doctor because you had a backache that hurt you so much you couldn't do your work (housework) properly. Which one of these would it be most important for the doctor to do? (*HAND RESPONDENT REVERSE SIDE OF CARD*)

A. Get you back to your usual activities (work, housework, etc.) as soon as possible 56-1

B. Make sure you have nothing serious 2

C. Make you feel better right away 3

D. Find out exactly what illness you have, even if this takes some time 4

E. Listen to your problems that may be making you sick 5

F. Teach you how to take care of your illness 6

Don't know 7

16. In general, when you're not feeling well, do you usually see a doctor right away; or do you wait a while, to see if it will go away; or do you usually put off seeing a doctor as long as you possibly can?

See doctor right away	57-1
Wait a while	2
Put off as long as possible	3
Don't know	4

17. Now here is a list of health conditions that people sometimes have. I'll read each one, and I'd like you to tell me if you think a person should see a doctor about it immediately, or should take care of it himself unless it keeps up or gets worse, or if he should just leave it alone.

First, how about a bad cough for several weeks — Should a person see a doctor about it right away, or should he take care of it himself unless it keeps up or gets worse, or should he just leave it alone? (*Continue through list*)

	See Doctor	Care Self	Leave Alone	Don't Know
A. Bad cough for several weeks	58-1	2	3	4
B. Diarrhea or constipation for a couple of days	59-1	2	3	4
C. Frequent headaches	60-1	2	3	4
D. Coughing up blood	61-1	2	3	4
E. Feeling tired all the time, no special reason	62-1	2	3	4
F. Feeling very depressed and blue	63-1	2	3	4
G. An unusual lump on the body	64-1	2	3	4
H. Shortness of breath	65-1	2	3	4
I. Sore throat, running nose, for a couple of days	66-1	2	3	4
J. Pain in the chest	67-1	2	3	4

18. Now here is a list of reasons that people sometimes give for not seeing a doctor when perhaps they should. Thinking back over your own experience, I'd like you to tell me which ones have ever kept you from seeing a doctor when perhaps you should have.

For instance, "I didn't know any really good doctor" — has that ever made you put off seeing a doctor? (*Continue through list, repeating "Has that ever made you put off seeing a doctor when perhaps you should have?"*)

	Yes	No	Don't Know
A. I didn't know any really good doctor	68-1	2	3
B. I didn't want to spend the money on a doctor unless I had to	69-1	2	3
C. Travelling in the city is such a problem	70-1	2	3
D. I don't like to bother the doctor unless it's necessary	71-1	2	3
E. I didn't think the doctor could help me any	72-1	2	3

	Yes	No	Don't Know
F. The doctor might want to put me in a hospital	73-1	2	3
G. I was too busy to see a doctor; I didn't have time	74-1	2	3
H. ASK ONLY IF CHILDREN UNDER 18 IN CASE: It's hard to go when I have the children to look after	75-1	2	3

76-	77-	78-	79-	80-

19. We're interested in how people feel about getting general physical check-ups. Suppose you were offered a free physical examination next week. Would you certainly go, probably go, or probably not go?

Certainly go	6-1
Probably go	2*
Probably not go	3**
Don't know	4*

*A. IF "PROBABLY GO" OR "DON'T KNOW": What would it depend on? (What sort of difficulties might you have?)

7-

8-

**B. IF "PROBABLY NOT GO": Why not?

9-

10-

20. ASK ONLY IF CHILDREN UNDER 18 IN CASE: Suppose you were offered a free physical examination for your children next week. Would you certainly take them, probably take them, or probably not take them?

Certainly take them	11-1
Probably take them	2*
Probably not take them	3**
Don't know	4*

*A. IF "PROBABLY TAKE THEM" OR "DON'T KNOW": What would it depend on? (What sort of difficulties might you have?)

12-

13-

**B. IF "PROBABLY NOT TAKE THEM": Why not?

14-

15-

---

21. We're interested in learning more about how people use doctors and clinics. Here are some conditions which usually need medical attention. Please tell me for each one where you would go – that is, would you *call a doctor, go to a clinic, or go to an emergency room?*

	Doctor	Clinic	Emerg. Room	Don't Know	Other (Explain)
A. Frequent stomach upsets	16-1	2	3	4	5
B. Varicose veins	17-1	2	3	4	5
C. A broken arm	18-1	2	3	4	5
D. Nervousness	19-1	2	3	4	5
E. If you thought you might have heart trouble	20-1	2	3	4	5
F. Troublesome boils	21-1	2	3	4	5
G. If you felt sick all over	22-1	2	3	4	5
H. If you were spitting blood	23-1	2	3	4	5
I. Itching skin that won't clear up	24-1	2	3	4	5
J. A fever of 105	25-1	2	3	4	5
K. Couldn't sleep because of worry	26-1	2	3	4	5
L. Unexplained weight loss over several months	27-1	2	3	4	5

---

22. Now here are some things people say about *hospitals.* When I say each one, I want you to tell me *which* hospital or hospitals in New York City seem that way to you. It doesn't matter if you haven't been there yourself – you may have heard other people talk about them.

Now which hospital seems to you *easy to get to? (Continue through list, writing in all comments verbatim)*

A. Easy to get to?

28-
29-

B. Good, but too far away?

30-
31-

C. Has the best doctors?　　　　　　　　　　　　　　　32-
　　　　　　　　　　　　　　　　　　　　　　　　　　　　33-

D. Keeps you waiting much too long?　　　　　　　　34-
　　　　　　　　　　　　　　　　　　　　　　　　　　　　35-

E. Only for rich people?　　　　　　　　　　　　　　　36-
　　　　　　　　　　　　　　　　　　　　　　　　　　　　37-

F. Overcrowded?　　　　　　　　　　　　　　　　　　38-
　　　　　　　　　　　　　　　　　　　　　　　　　　　　39-

G. Not enough doctors and nurses?　　　　　　　　　40-
　　　　　　　　　　　　　　　　　　　　　　　　　　　　41-

H. Friendly?　　　　　　　　　　　　　　　　　　　　42-
　　　　　　　　　　　　　　　　　　　　　　　　　　　　43-

I. Gloomy, or dirty?　　　　　　　　　　　　　　　　44-
　　　　　　　　　　　　　　　　　　　　　　　　　　　　45-

J. Doesn't treat you like a person?　　　　　　　　　46-
　　　　　　　　　　　　　　　　　　　　　　　　　　　　47-

---

23. IF NEW YORK HOSPITAL MENTIONED ANYWHERE ABOVE:

You mentioned New York Hospital is (*see above*). What *else* do you know, or have you heard, about New York Hospital? Anything else? (*Probe and record fully*)

48-

49-

---

24. IF NO MENTION OF NEW YORK HOSPITAL ANYWHERE IN Q. 22:

Have you ever heard of New York
Hospital?　　　　　　　　　　　　　Yes　　　　　　50-1*
　　　　　　　　　　　　　　　　　　No　　　　　　　　2

*A. IF "YES": What do you know, or what have you heard, about New York Hospital? (Anything else?)

51-

52-

25. Have you, or anyone else you know, ever had an experience with any hospital that gave you a poor opinion of that hospital?

Yes	53-1*
No	2

*IF "YES", ASK BOTH "A" & "B"

A. Who was that?

Self	54-1
Spouse	2
Other relative	3
Friend, acquaintance	4

B. What happened?

55-

56-

C. Was that in New York City? (*IF YES*) What hospital was that?

57-

58-

IF "USE HEALTH QUESTIONNAIRE" BOX IS CHECKED ON

FACE SHEET, COMPLETE HEALTH QUESTIONNAIRE

NOW BEFORE GOING ON TO Q. 26.

IF "USE HEALTH QUESTIONNAIRE" BOX IS NOT CHECKED,

GO ON WITH Q. 26.

---

26. And now a question about things in general. During the next couple of years, do you think most people in this country, in general, will be better off financially, about the same as they are now, or worse off?

Better off	59-1
About same	2
Worse off	3
Don't know	4

---

27. And how about you yourself (and your family) – During the next couple of years, do you think you will be better off financially, about the same as you are now, or worse off?

Better off	60-1
About same	2
Worse off	3
Don't know	4

28. Many people say they can live only from one day to another at this time. Do you think this way too, or do you believe you can make plans for the future?

One day to another	61-1
Can plan for future	2
Don't know	3

29. How long have you been living at this address?

_____ 62-
(specify years, months or days, as case may be)

30. A. What is your religious preference?

Protestant	63-1*
Catholic	2
Jewish	3
Other (specify)	4
None	5

*B. IF "PROTESTANT": What denomination?

C. How often do you attend church (synagogue) services?

Once a week or more	64-1
1-3 times a month	2
Less than once a month	3
Never	4

D. Quite apart from church (synagogue) going, how important would you say religion is to you - very important, fairly important, or not important at all?

Very important	65-1
Fairly important	2
Not important at all	3
Don't know	4

A. NAME OF RESPONDENT:

_____

B. How long did this interview
take?

66-

_____

C. RESPONDENT'S ATTITUDE
WAS: (Circle one)

Friendly, eager	67-1
Cooperative	2
Passive, indifferent	3
Hostile, suspicious	4

_____

D. RESPONDENT IS: (Circle one)

White	68-1
Puerto Rican "A"	2
Puerto Rican "B"	3
Puerto Rican "C"	4
Negro	5
Other (Specify)	6

_____

E. LANGUAGE USED IN
INTERVIEW:

English, no difficulty	69-1
English, some difficulty	2
English, very hard to com-	
municate	3
Spanish	4
Other language (specify)	5

_____

F. Was communication with this
respondent difficult for any
reason (besides language)?

Yes (Explain)	69-8
No	9

_____

G. Does respondent live alone or
with others?

Lives alone	70-1
With others	2

H. Was any other person present
while you were conducting
the interview?

Yes	71-1*
No	2

*A. IF "YES": Do you think
this affected his answers
in any way? (If yes,
explain)

_____

I. Do you believe this respondent thought you were con-
nected with the Welfare
Department, or New York
Hospital, or some other
agency besides NORC?

Yes	72-1*
No	2
Don't know	3

*IF "YES", ANSWER "1"
& "2"

1. Who did he think sent
you?

73-

2. Do you think this
affected his anwers in any
way? (If yes, explain)

74-

_____

J. INTERVIEWER'S SIGNA-
TURE:

_____

K. DATE OF INTERVIEW:

75-

AFTER CHECKING THIS

INTERVIEW FOR RECORD-

ING ERRORS OR OMISSIONS

ATTACH FACE SHEET TO

FIRST PAGE

_____

76-   77-   78-   79-   80-

280

NORC
438

HEALTH QUESTIONNAIRE – ILLNESS LIST

If there is a Spouse in this case, fill out one copy of this "Illness List" for the Respondent and a second copy for the Spouse. Interview the Respondent about Spouse (unless the latter is easily available), rephrasing all questions in terms of "Does your (husband, wife) have . . .Has (he or she) ever had. . .?" etc.

NORC CASE NO.	THIS ILLNESS LIST REFERS TO: *(enter name of Respondent or Spouse)*	Circle one:	
		Respondent	9-1
		Spouse	2

1. I'm going to read you a list of illnesses, and I would like you to tell me for each one whether or not you have it now. The first one is asthma. Do you have asthma now?

> IF YES: CIRCLE APPROPRIATE CODE 1 BELOW
> IF DK: PROBE "Has a doctor ever told you you have asthma?"
> IF NO: ASK "A" AND CIRCLE EITHER 5 OR 6

A. IF "NO": Have you ever had asthma?

REPEAT FOR EACH ILLNESS IN TURN. IGNORE "Doctor checks at intake COLUMN

	Has Now	Doctor Checks At Intake		Not Now But Has Had	Never
Asthma	10-1	2	3	4 — 5	6
Allergies (e.g., rash, hay fever)	11-1	2	3	4 — 5	6
Sinus trouble (stuffiness with pain in the face)	12-1	2	3	4 — 5	6
Tuberculosis	13-1	2	3	4 — 5	6
Rheumatic fever or growing pains	14-1	2	3	4 — 5	6
Heart trouble	15-1	2	3	4 — 5	6
Stroke (a clot in the brain with paralysis)	16-1	2	3	4 — 5	6
High blood pressure (hypertension)	17-1	2	3	4 — 5	6
Hardening of the arteries, arteriosclerosis	18-1	2	3	4 — 5	6
IF YES: What part of the body?					
Varicose veins, swollen veins	19-1	2	3	4 — 5	6
Stomach ulcers, peptic ulcers	20-1	2	3	4 — 5	6
Liver disease, yellow jaundice	21-1	2	3	4 — 5	6
Gallstones	22-1	2	3	4 — 5	6
Cancer	23-1	2	3	4 — 5	6

Q. 1 CONTINUED

	Has Now	Doctor Checks at intake			Not Now But Has Had	Never Had
Rupture, hernia	24-1	2	3	4 __	5	6
Parasites or worms	25-1	2	3	4 __	5	6
Kidney or bladder disease	26-1	2	3	4 __	5	6
Thyroid disease or goiter	27-1	2	3	4 __	5	6
Diabetes (sugar)	28-1	2	3	4 __	5	6
Severe anemia, thin blood	29-1	2	3	4 __	5	6
Syphilis, bad blood	30-1	2	3	4 __	5	6
Gonorrhea, clap	31-1	2	3	4 __	5	6
Arthritis	32-1	2	3	4 __	5	6
Hemorrhoids, piles	33-1	2	3	4 __	5	6
Epilepsy, falling out spells	34-1	2	3	4 __	5	6
Do you suffer from nerves?	35-1	2	3	4 __	5	6
Any serious lung trouble (causing trouble breathing)? IF YES: What is (was) it?	36-1	2	3	4 __	5	6
A tumor IF YES: Where is (was) it?	37-1	2	3	4 __	5	6
WOMEN: Women's trouble (of ovary or womb)	38-1	2	3	4 __	5	6
MEN: Prostate gland trouble	39-1	2	3	4 __	5	6

Do you now have any other illnesses we haven't mentioned?
(*Write in below*)

Doctor's Diagnostic Impression at Intake

Date_____.

_____
_____
_____
_____
_____

		Yes	No
2.	Do you have trouble with your eyes?	62-1	R
	Do you have trouble with your hearing?	2	R
	Do you have cavities or decay in any of your teeth?	3	R
	Do you have any other trouble with your teeth?	4	R
	Do you often have severe headaches?	5	R
	Have you had a bad cough for several weeks?	6	R
	In the last year, have you coughed up blood?	7	R
	Do you have a pain in the chest?	8	R
	Do you have difficulty breathing?	63-1	R
	Are your ankles often very swollen?	2	R
	Do you suffer from indigestion?	3	R
	Have you lost a lot of weight recently, without dieting?	4	R

Q. 2 CONTINUED

	Yes	No
Do you often vomit?	5	R
Have you begun to have diarrhea lately?	6	R
Have you begun to be constipated lately?	7	R
In the last year, have your bowel movements been bloody at times?	8	R
Have you had any trouble with urination (passing water)?	9	R
In the last year, have you ever passed blood when urinating?	0	R
Have you noticed any unusual lumps on your body?	64-1	R
Do you have any kind of skin trouble, e.g., skin irritation, rash, sores	2	R
Do you often have back aches?	3	R
Are your joints ever painfully swollen?	4	R
Do you have trouble sleeping?	5	R
Is your appetite usually poor?	6	R
Are you continually troubled with aches and pains?	7	R
When you are sick, do you often have to go to bed?	8	R
Do you feel tired all the time for no special reason?	9	R
Have you recently been very depressed and blue?	0	R

WOMEN:			
Have your menstrual periods been irregular or have you had bleeding between periods?	65-1	2
Have you often had to lie down when your periods came on?	66-1	2
Do you have a constant vaginal discharge or itching?	67-1	2

3. Have you ever had any operations? Yes 68-1*
   No 2

*IF "YES", ASK "A", THEN "B" & "C" ABOUT EACH

A. What kinds of operations were they? Any others?	B. When was that?	C. In what hospital was that?
_____ 69-	70-	_____71-
_____		_____72-
_____		

4. Have you ever had any serious injury?   Yes   73-1*

                                                            No   2

*IF "YES", ASK "A" & "B"

| A. | B. |
| What kind of injury was that? (Any others?) | When was that? |

_____ 74-   _____ 75-

_____   _____

_____   _____

5. A. Do you have any illnesses or health conditions that interfere with your usual work? (*Circle on A under NO or YES below*)

   B. Does any illness or health condition interfere with your daily activities in the home, other than work -- such as dressing yourself, getting around the house, and so on? (*Circle on "B"*)

   C. Does any illness or health condition interfere with your traveling around the city, such as walking, taking the bus or subway? (*Circle on "C"*)

   D. Does any illness or health condition interfere with any other activities you might engage in, such as going to visit your family or friends or local community groups? (*Circle on "D"*)

   E. FOR EACH "YES" CIRCLED BELOW: Would you say the condition interferes with your (A, B, C or D) a great deal, or some, or only a little?

	NO	YES	Great Deal	Some	Only a Little
A. Work or housework	76-1	R	2	3	4
B. Other daily activity	77-1	R	2	3	4
C. Traveling around	78-1	R	3	3	4
D. Social life	79-1	R	2	3	4

INTERVIEWER'S SIGNATURE:_____ DATE_____

NORC:438

HEALTH QUESTIONNAIRE – UTILIZATION

CASE NO._____

CHECK YOUR FACE SHEET

IF SPOUSE IN CASE, ASK: What is your (spouse's) name? (Record under "Spouse" below)
IF CHILDREN UNDER 18 IN CASE, ASK: What are the names of the children under 18? (Record full name of each child below)

1. Have (either of, any of) you ever been a patient at (*each hospital below*)?
   IF NO, CIRCLE "NO" ON APPROPRIATE LINE
   IF YES, PROBE IF NECESSARY TO FIND OUT WHO (and "Anyone else"?), THEN ASK: About when were you (was he/she) last there as a patient?
   ENTER DATE IN APPROPRIATE COLUMN. IF DATE IS 1960 OR 1961, PROBE FOR MONTH. THEN GO ON TO NEXT HOSPITAL.

	RESPONDENT	SPOUSE	CHILD	CHILD	CHILD	CHILD
01 Metropolitan	NO					
02 Bellevue	NO					
03 Mount Sinai	NO					
04 New York Eye & Ear	NO					
05 St. Vincent's	NO					
06 N.Y. Hospital – Cornell	NO					
07 Columbia Presbyt. (Medical Center)	NO					
08 Flower-Fifth Ave.	NO					
09 Lenox Hill	NO					
10 Harlem	NO					

2. Have (either, any of) you ever been a patient at any other hospitals in New York City that I didn't mention? IF NO, CIRCLE "NO". IF YES, ASK: What other hospital? Any others? AND RECORD AT LEFT BELOW. PROBE FOR WHO USED THEM IF NECESSARY, THEN RECORD *DATE* OF LAST USE IN APPROPRIATE COLUMNS BELOW. IF 1960 OR 1961, PROBE FOR MONTH.

NO

_____

_____

3. Have you (either, any of you) ever been a patient at a mental hospital anywhere? IF NO, CIRCLE "NO". IF YES, ASK: What hospital was that? Any others? AND RECORD AT LEFT BELOW, PROBE FOR WHO PATIENT WAS IF NECESSARY, THEN RECORD DATE OF LAST USE OF HOSPITAL IN APPROPRIATE COLUMN BELOW, IF 1960 OR 1961, PROBE FOR MONTH.

NO

_____

_____

4. REFER TO Qs. 1, 2 & 3 AND RECORD BELOW THE NAMES OF ALL HOSPITALS USED *DURING THE LAST TWELVE MONTHS*, AND THE NAMES OF ALL PERSONS USING ANY HOSPITAL DURING THE LAST TWELVE MONTHS.

A. Now I want to ask you about the last twelve months – that is, since (month) last year.
   You mentioned that (you or name of individual) had been in (name of) hospital during the last 12 months. Was (person) *a bed patient* there during that period? IF YES: For about how many days was (person) a bed patient? (RECORD NO. OF DAYS ON "A" LINE IN APPROPRIATE COLUMN)

B. Was (person) *a clinic patient* there at any time during the last twelve months? IF YES: About how many times did (person) use the clinic at (name of) hospital? (RECORD ON "B" LINE IN PROPER COLUMN)

C. Did (person) ever use *the emergency room* at (name of) hospital during the last twelve months?
   IF YES: About how many times? (RECORD ON "C" LINE IN APPROPRIATE COLUMN)

REPEAT "A", "B", & "C" FOR EACH *OTHER* HOSPITAL THAT PERSON USED, IF MORE THAN ONE. *THEN GO ON TO NEXT PERSON.*

NAME OF HOSPITAL	RESPONDENT	SPOUSE	CHILD	CHILD	CHILD
	A: ____ days B: ____ times C: ____ times	A: ____ days B: ____ times C: ____ times	A: ____ days B: ____ times C: ____ times	A: ____ days B: ____ times C: ____ times	A: ____ days B: ____ times C: ____ times
	A: ____ days B: ____ times C: ____ times	A: ____ days B: ____ times C: ____ times	A: ____ days B: ____ times C: ____ times	A: ____ days B: ____ times C: ____ times	A: ____ days B: ____ times C: ____ times
	A: ____ days B: ____ times C: ____ times	A: ____ days B: ____ times C: ____ times	A: ____ days B: ____ times C: ____ times	A: ____ days B: ____ times C: ____ times	A: ____ days B: ____ times C: ____ times
	A: ____ days B: ____ times C: ____ times	A: ____ days B: ____ times C: ____ times	A: ____ days B: ____ times C: ____ times	A: ____ days B: ____ times C: ____ times	A: ____ days B: ____ times C: ____ times
	A: ____ days B: ____ times C: ____ times	A: ____ days B: ____ times C: ____ times	A: ____ days B: ____ times C: ____ times	A: ____ days B: ____ times C: ____ times	A: ____ days B: ____ times C: ____ times

5. During the last twelve months, have you (either, any of you) been to a clinic *not* in a hospital, like a health clinic or welfare clinic? IF NO, CIRCLE "NO" BELOW.
IF YES, PROBE FOR WHO, IF NECESSARY, AND ASK: How many times did (each person) go to this kind of clinic? RECORD BELOW IN APPROPRIATE COLUMN.

6. During the last twelve months, have you (either, any of you) seen a doctor *in his office*? IF NO, CIRCLE "NO".
IF YES: PROBE FOR WHO, IF NECESSARY, AND ASK: How many times did (each person) visit a doctor in his office? RECORD BELOW IN APPROPRIATE COLUMN.

7. During the last twelve months, did a doctor ever *come to your home*? IF NO, CIRCLE "NO".
IF YES: PROBE FOR WHOM HE VISITED, IF NECESSARY, AND ASK: How many times did a doctor visit (each person) at your home? RECORD BELOW IN APPROPRIATE COLUMN.

8. A. And during the last twelve months, did you (yourself) see a dentist, nurse, or anyone else about your health? IF NO, CIRCLE "NO" UNDER RESPONDENT. IF YES, ASK: Whom did you see? RECORD BELOW UNDER RESPONDENT.

B. REPEAT "A" FOR EACH OTHER FAMILY MEMBER IN CASE.

	RESPONDENT	SPOUSE	CHILD	CHILD	CHILD	CHILD
5. CLINIC NOT IN HOSP. NO	times	times	times	times	times	times
6. DOCTOR IN OFFICE NO	times	times	times	times	times	times
7. DR. VISIT AT HOME NO	times	times	times	times	times	times

288

8. OTHER

	NO		NO		NO		NO		NO
Dentist		1		1		1		1		1
Nurse		2		2		2		2		2
Other (Who?)									

NOW GO BACK TO Q.26 OF ATTITUDE QUESTIONNAIRE

INTERVIEWER: _____

DATE: _____

ENTER CASE NO.

NATIONAL OPINION RESEARCH CENTER
University of Chicago

H E A L T H C A R E S T U D Y

A. First tell me, how long have you been
living at this address? _____

(specify years, months or days)

IF LESS THAN INTERVAL SINCE FIRST INTERVIEW, ASK:

(1) Where were you living before that? _____

(2) How long had you been living there? _____

B. Now I need a list of all the people who live in this household. (LIST RESPOND-
ENT ON FIRST LINE.) Besides yourself, who else lives here? Let's take them in
order of age. (CONTINUE LISTING ALL HOUSEHOLD MEMBERS.)

C. Have we missed any children or babies or anyone else who lives here -- anyone
away traveling, in a hospital, visiting somewhere, or in an institution? (IF YES,
ADD TO LISTING)

D. Has anyone else lived in this household since (date of first interview), who isn't
living here now? (IF YES, ADD NAME TO LISTING)

E. FOR EACH PERSON LISTED, RECORD RELATIONSHIP TO RESPONDENT,
AGE, SEX, MARITAL STATUS (M-S-W-D-Sep) AND NUMBER OF MONTHS
IN HOUSEHOLD SINCE FIRST INTERVIEW.

Last Name	First Name	Relation to Resp.	Age	Sex	Marital Status	No. of Months

HAVE ALL CASE MEMBERS LISTED ON FACE SHEET OPPOSITE BEEN
LISTED ABOVE?
IF NOT, RECORD PRESENT ADDRESS OF EACH ABSENT CASE MEMBER
ON FACE SHEET.

HAVE ANY NEW BABIES BEEN BORN TO A MOTHER IN THE CASE
SINCE FIRST INTERVIEW?
IF YES, ADD THE CHILD TO THE LIST OF CASE MEMBERS ON FACE
SHEET OPPOSITE.

1. A. Would you say your own health, in general, is excellent, good, fair, or poor?

   B. IF SPOUSE IN CASE: How about the health of your (spouse) -- In general, would you rate it as excellent, good, fair, or poor?

   C. IF CHILDREN IN CASE: How about the health of the child(ren), in general?

	A. Self	B. Spouse	C. Children
Excellent	6-1*	7-1	8-1
Good	2*	2	2
Fair	3**	3	3
Poor	4**	4	4
Don't know	5**	5	5

*D. IF OWN HEALTH "EXCELLENT" OR "GOOD": Are there any small things that bother you? (What?)

9-

10-

**E. IF OWN HEALTH "FAIR", "POOR" OR "DON'T KNOW": What are the main things that bother you? (Anything else?)

11-

12-

   F. IF SPOUSE IN CASE: How about your (spouse's) health – is there anything bothering (him, her)?

13-

14-

   G. IF CHILDREN IN CASE: Are there any particular things about your child(ren)'s health which bother you?

15-

16-

NOW MAKE OUT A UTILIZATION SUPPLEMENT FOR EACH CASE MEMBER, INCLUDING ANY NEW BABIES ADDED TO LIST ON BACK OF FACE SHEET AND INCLUDING ANY CASE MEMBERS NOW DECEASED.

2. Since (date of last interview), has any visiting nurse come to your home?

                        Yes   R*
                        No   Z

*IF YES, ASK BOTH "A" & "B"

  A. How many times, altogether, did a
     visiting nurse come to your home
     since (date)?   _____

  B. IF MORE THAN ONE CASE
     MEMBER: And which of you did
     she come to see?   _____

---

3. Since (date), how many times have you talked to a doctor *on the telephone*, about an illness or injury of your own or anyone else we've talked about? (*Explore reasons and outcome of phone conversations and record verbatim.*)

                                           17-

                                           18-

---

4. Since (date), was there any time that a hospital did not give you (or anyone else we've talked about) medical care when you asked for it?

                        Yes   R*
                        No   Z

*IF YES, ASK "A" & "B" & "C"

  A. What hospital was that?   19-

  B. What happened? (PROBE: Did they   20-
     send you somewhere else? Did you go?)

                                       21-

  C. Any other times? (*If Yes, repeat A & B)*   22-

                                       23-

---

5. How about private doctors – Was there any time that a private doctor did not give you (or anyone else we've talked about) medical care himself when you asked for it?

                        Yes   R*
                        No   Z

*IF YES, ASK "A" & "B"

292

A. What happened? (PROBE: Did he send you somewhere else? Did you go?)

24-

B. Any other times? (*If Yes, repeat A*)   25-

26-

CHECK PAGES 1 & 2 OF *EACH UTILIZATION SUPPLEMENT* FOR ALL *HOSPITALS* USED, AND RECORD HOSPITAL NAMES BELOW. THEN ASK Q. 6.

IF NO HOSPITALS USED, CHECK BOX AND SKIP TO TOP OF PAGE 6.   ☐

---

6. A. Now you said (you and/or name) went to (name of hospital). Taking every-thing into consideration, what were some of the things you liked most about the care and treatment (you and/or name) got there?

B. And what were some of the things you didn't like so much about the care and treatment (you and/or name) got there -- even little things?

REPEAT QUESTION 6 FOR EACH HOSPITAL LISTED.

LIKED MOST		LIKED LEAST
	27-	
(name of hospital)	28-	
2 9		
3 0		
3 1		
3 2		
3 3		
3 4		

LIKED MOST   LIKED LEAST

	35-	
(name of hospital)	36-	
3 7		
3 8		
3 9		
4 0		
4 1		
4 2		

	43-	
(name of hospital)	44-	
4 5		
4 6		
4 7		
4 8		
4 9		
5 0		

7. ASK ONLY IF TWO OR MORE HOSPITALS LISTED IN Q. 6.

Some people (families) use only one hospital for all their medical care, while others use more than one. I see that you (your family) have used (*name each hospital listed*).

How is it that you went to more than one hospital for your medical care?

51-

52-

REFER TO *Q. 3* (HOSPITAL CLINICS OR EMERGENCY ROOMS) AND *Q. 7* (PRIVATE DOCTORS) ON *EACH UTILIZATION SUPPLEMENT.*

IF BOTH PRIVATE DOCTOR AND HOSPITAL CLINIC OR EMERGENCY ROOM USED, ASK Q. 8.

IF ONLY ONE OR NEITHER USED, CHECK BOX AND OMIT Q. 8. ☐

---

8. I see that you (your family) went to (*name of hospital clinic(s) and /or emergency room(s)*), and also to a private doctor(s).

   How is it that you used both a private doctor and hospital facilities:

   53-

   54-

HOSPITALS USED SINCE 1957
(from back of Face Sheet) _____

HOSPITALS USED LAST YEAR
(from Q. 6) _____

IF MORE THAN ONE HOSPITAL LISTED ABOVE, ASK Q. 9.

IF ONLY ONE HOSPITAL LISTED ABOVE, SKIP TO Q. 10.

IF NO HOSPITAL LISTED ABOVE AND ANY MEDICAL CARE LAST YEAR, SKIP TO Q. 11.

IF NO HOSPITAL LISTED ABOVE AND NO MEDICAL CARE LAST YEAR, SKIP TO Q. 12.

---

9. IF ANY HOSPITAL LISTED ON FIRST LINE ABOVE: Last year when you were interviewed you (your family) had been using (*hospital(s) on first line above*).

   IF ANY HOSPITAL LISTED ON SECOND LINE ABOVE: This year I notice you used *(hospital(s) on second line above).*

   A. Which hospitals do you think you will keep on using if you need   55-
      medical care next year?   56-
      57-
      58-

   B. Are you likely to use any other hospitals – either any of these or any
      we haven't mentioned? (IF YES) Which?   59-
      60-
      61-

C. IF ONLY ONE MENTIONED IN "A" & "B": Why will you probably use (*hospital named in "A"*) rather than (*other(s) listed above*)?

63-

D. IF MORE THAN ONE MENTIONED IN "A" & "B": Under what circumstances would you be likely to use (*each hospital named in "A" & "B"*)

64-

65-

NOW SKIP TO Q. 11.

---

10. IF ONLY ONE HOSPITAL EVER USED: If you need medical care next year, do you think you will keep on using (*name of hospital*), or will you go to some other hospital?

Keep using same	R
Go to other	Z*
Don't know	W

   *A. IF "GO TO OTHER": Which one?   66-

67-

---

11. Altogether, would you say the medical care you (your family) got this past year was better, about the same, or worse than the medical care you got the year before?

Better	68-1*
About the same	2
Worse	3*
Don't know	4

   *A. IF BETTER OR WORSE; In what way was it (better, worse)?

69-

---

12. ASK EVERYONE: In general, when you're not feeling well, do you usually see a doctor right away; or do you wait a while, to see if it will go away; or do you usually put off seeing a doctor as long as you possibly can?

See doctor right away	70-1
Wait a while	2
Put off as long as possible	3
Don't know	4

13. If you could choose, and it didn't cost you anything, would you rather go to a *hospital* clinic or emergency room, or would you rather see a private doctor?

Clinic or emergency room	71-1*
Private doctor	2*
Don't know	3

  *A. IF "CLINIC OR EMERGENCY ROOM" OR "PRIVATE DOCTOR": Why?

72-

73-

---

14. When you go to a clinic, how important is it that you see the same doctor each time -- is that very important to you, fairly important, or not important at all?

Very important	74-1
Fairly important	2
Not important	3
Don't know	4

    75-   76-   77-   78-   79-   80-

---

15. Here are some things people sometimes say about doctors. I'd like to know whether you personally think they are true of *most* doctors, or not. For example (*READ "A"*). Do you think that's true of most doctors, or not? (*Continue through list, circling one code for each.*)

	True of most	Not True	Don't Know
A. They don't give you a chance to tell them exactly what your trouble is	6-1	2	3
B. They don't take enough personal interest in you	7-1	2	3
C. Doctors want you to come back for additional visits even if you don't need to	8-1	2	3
D. They don't tell you enough about your condition; they don't explain just what the trouble is	9-1	2	3
E. Doctors give better care to their private patients than to their clinic patients	10-1	2	3
F. They tell you there's nothing wrong with you when you know there is	11-1	2	3
G. Doctors rush too much when they examine you	12-1	2	3
H. Doctors are very understanding people	13-1	2	3
I. Doctors go out of their way to help you	14-1	2	3

16. If you had a chance to talk to a doctor for half an hour, at no cost to you, are there any things about your own health that you'd like to ask him right now?

Yes	15-1*
No	2**
Don't know	3

*A. IF YES: What sort of things would you ask him about right now? (Anything else?) (*Record below*)

**B. IF NO: Why is that? 16-

17-

18-

---

17. ASK ONLY IF SPOUSE OR CHILDREN IN CASE:
Are there any particular things you'd like to ask a doctor about the health of other members of your family right now?

Yes	19-1*
No	2**
Don't know	3

*A. IF YES: What sort of things? (Anything else?) *Record below and specify person if applicable*)

20-

**B. IF NO: Why is that?

21-

22-

---

18. If you suddenly needed a doctor at night or on a Sunday, what would you do? (*Do NOT read answer categories*)

Phone doctor	23-1*
Send someone to get a doctor	2*
Call police or ambulance	3*
Go to an emergency room	4*
Other (*specify*)	5*
Don't know	6

IF "DON'T KNOW", SKIP TO Q. 19.

*A. How much trouble do you think you would have getting medical care that way (*Repeat response to Question 18 if necessary*), if you suddenly got sick at night or on a Sunday – a great deal of trouble, some trouble, or not trouble at all?

Great deal	24-1**
Some	2**
No trouble at all	3**
Don't inow	4

**B. UNLESS DON'T KNOW TO "A": Why is that?

---

19. We're interested in learning more about how people use doctors and clinics. Here are some conditions which usually need medical attention. Please tell me for each one where you would go – that is, would you *call a doctor, go to a clinic,* or *go to an emergency room?*

	Doctor	Clinic	Emergency Room	Don't Know	Other (Explain)
A. Frequent stomach upsets	26-1*	2	3	4	5
B. Varicose veins	27-1*	2	3	4	5
C. A broken arm	28-1*	2	3	4	5
D. Nervousness	29-1*	2	3	4	5
E. If you thought you might have heart trouble	30-1*	2	3	4	5
F. Troublesome boils	31-1*	2	3	4	5
G. If you felt sick all over	32-1*	2	3	4	5
H. If you were spitting blood	33-1*	2	3	4	5
I. Itching skin that won't clear up	34-1*	2	3	4	5
J. A fever of 105	35-1*	2	3	4	5
K. Couldn't sleep because of worry	36-1*	2	3	4	5
L. Unexplained weight loss over several months	37-1*	2	3	4	5

*M. IF "1" CIRCLED ON ANY ITEM: You said you would call a doctor for (*items coded 1*). Would that be a private doctor or a doctor from a clinic?

Private	R
Clinic	Z
Other (*specify*)	W

---

38

20. Now here are some things people say about *hospitals*. When I say each one, I want you to tell me *which* hospital or hospitals in New York City seem that way to you. It doesn't matter if you haven't been there yourself – you may have heard other people talk about them.

Now which hospital seems to you *easy to get to*? (*CONTINUE THROUGH LIST, WRITING IN ALL COMMENTS VERBATIM*)

A. Easy to get to?

B. Good, but too far away?

41

C. Has the best doctors?   43-

44-

D. Keeps you waiting much too long?   45-

46-

E. Only for rich people   47-

48-

F. Overcrowded?   49-

50-

G. Not enough doctors and nurses?   51-

52-

H. Friendly?   53-

54-

I. Gloomy, or dirty?   55-

56-

J. Doesn't treat you like a person?   57-

58-

---

21. And now here are some things that people say about going to doctors, and I'd like to know how strongly you agree or disagree with each one. Just tell me which statement on this card comes closest to your own feeling. (*HAND RESPONDENT WHITE CARD*)

A. Going to a doctor is a sign of weakness. A person should be able to take care of himself.

B. Common sense goes a whole lot further in taking care of your health than doctors with all their book learning.

C. Doctors pry into your personal life and ask you questions that are none of their business.

	A. Sign of Weakness	B. Common Sense	C. Doctors Pry
Agree strongly	59-1	60-1	61-1
Agree somewhat	2	2	2
Uncertain	3	3	3
Disagree somewhat	4	4	4
Disagree strongly	5	5	5

Up to now we've been asking you questions about your health. Now I'd like to ask you just a few different questions.

22. During the next couple of years, do you think most people in this country, in general, will be better off financially, about the same as they are now, or worse off?

Better off	62-1
About the same	2
Worse off	3
Don't know	4

23. And how about you yourself (and your family) -- During the next couple of years, do you think *you* will be better off financially, about the same as you are now, or worse off?

Better off	63-1
About the same	2
Worse off	3
Don't know	4

24. Many people say they can live only from one day to another at this time. Do you think this way too, or do you believe you can make plans for the future?

One day to another	64-1
Can plan for future	2
Don't know	3

25. A. In what country was your father born? _____ 65-

    B. In what country was you mother born? _____ 66-

    IF EITHER BORN OUTSIDE U.S. MAINLAND:

    C. In what country were you born? _____ 67-

        IF RESPONDENT BORN OUTSIDE U.S. MAINLAND, ASK EITHER "D" OR "E"

    D. IF PUERTO RICO: How old were you when you
           came to the U.S. mainland?   _____
                                                                  68-

    E. IF FOREIGN BORN: How old were you when you
           came to this country?   _____

26. A. What is (was) your father's full name? _____

    B. What is (was) your mother's full name
       (before she was married)? _____

    IF SPOUSE IN CASE, ASK "C" & "D"

    C. What is (was) your (spouse's)
       father's full name? _____

    D. And what is (was) your (spouse's)
       mother's full name (before she
       was married)? _____

---

27. A. Do you feel you had a chance to get   Yes   69-1
       as much schooling as you wanted?   No   2

    B. How many years of school did you finish?

Never attended school	70-1	Completed 8 years	70-5
Completed 1-3 years	2	Completed 9-11 years	6
Completed 4-5 years	3	Completed 12 years	7
Completed 6-7 years	4	More than 12 years	8

---

28. And now would you give me the name of a relative or friend, outside the household, with whom you keep in touch. (This is just in case we want to reach you again in a year or so, and might not have your current address.)

PLEASE PRINT: _____
            (first name)   (last name)

Address_____ City & State _____

How related to you?_____

A. How long did this interview take?

71-

B. RESPONDENTS' ATTITUDE WAS: (*Circle one*):

Friendly, eager	72-1
Cooperative	2
Passive, indifferent	3
Hostile, suspicious	4

C. Do you believe this respondent thought you were connected with the Welfare Department or New York Hospital, or some other agency besides NORC?

Yes	73-1*
No	2
Don't know	3

*IF YES, ANSWER "1" & "2"

1. Who did he think sent you?

2. Do you think this affected his answers in any way? (*If yes, explain*)

D. Was any other person present while you were conducting the interview?

Yes	74-1*
No	2

*IF YES: Do you think this affected his answers in any way? (*If yes, explain*)

E. Was communication with this respondent difficult for any reason (besides language)?

Yes (*Explain*)	75-1
No	2

F. INTERVIEWER'S SIGNATURE:

G. DATE OF INTERVIEW:

76-

AFTER CHECKING THIS INTERVIEW FOR RECORDING ERRORS OR OMMISSIONS, ATTACH FACE SHEET TO FIRST PAGE.

77-   78-   79-   80-

NORC
455

HEALTH CARE STUDY

UTILIZATION SUPPLEMENT

NAME:·_____   CASE NO._____

Now I want to ask you some questions about any medical care that (you or name of case member) have had since the last time we talked with you on (date of first wave interview)

1. First, were (you, name) a *bed patient* in any hospital since (date of first interview)?

Yes	1*
No	2

*IF YES, ASK A-B-C

   A. What hospital was that? (*Record at bottom of page*)

   B. How many different times were (you, name) a bed patient in that hospital since (date)? (*Record name of hospital on SEPARATE LINE FOR EACH AD-MISSION*)

   C. Were (you, name) a bed patient in any other hospital since (date)?

     IF NO, GO ON TO Q. 2.

     IF YES, RECORD HOSPITAL NAME BELOW, ASK HOW MANY TIMES, AND THEN REPEAT A. 1-C

---

2. Were (you, name) a patient in any *mental* hospital since (date of first interview)?

Yes	1*
No	2

*IF YES, ASK A-B-C

   A. What hospital was that? (*Record below*)

   B. How many different times were (you, name) a patient in that hospital since (date)? (*Record name of hospital on SEPARATE LINE FOR EACH AD-MISSION*)

   C. Were (you, name) a patient in any other mental hospital since (date)?

     IF NO, GO ON TO Q. 3

     IF YES, RECORD HOSPITAL NAME BELOW, ASK HOW MANY TIMES, AND THEN REPEAT Q. 2-C

NAME:_____

| HOSPITAL | VERBATIM REMARKS (nature of condition, etc.) |

_____
_____
_____
_____
_____
_____
_____

3. Since (date of first interview) did (you, name) go to any *hospital or emergency room*?

Yes	1*
No	2

*IF YES, ASK FOLLOWING SERIES

A. At what hospital was that? (*Record below*)

B. Did you go to the clinic or to the emergency room?

    IF CLINIC: *Probe for exact name of clinic and ask to see clinic card number. Record below.*

    IF EMERGENCY ROOM: *Record "Emerg." below.*

    IF BOTH: *Use two lines below.*

C. Since (date), did (you, name) go to any other hospital clinic or emergency room?

    IF NO, GO ON TO "D" & "E"

    IF YES, RECORD HOSPITAL NAME BELOW, THEN REPEAT "B" & "C"

NOW ASK "D" & "E" SEPARATELY FOR EACH LINE BELOW

D. About how many times did (you, name) go to (name of clinic or emergency room) since (date of last interview)? (*Record below*)

E. And how many of those times did (you, name) actually see a doctor? (*Record below*)

NAME:_____

HOSPITAL CLINICS OR EMERGENCY ROOMS

Hospital	Name of Clinic or Emergency Room	Clinic Card Number	Total Number of Visits	No. Times Doctor Seen

4. Since (date of first interview), did (you, name) go to any clinic or health center *not in a hospital?*

Yes	1*
No	2

*IF YES: Which one? Any others? (*Record EXACT NAME AND ADDRESS below, or else record most accurate possible description and location of clinic*)

5. How about any of these kinds of clinics or health centers? (HAND CORRECT SIDE OF BLUE CARD) Since (date), did (you, name) go to any of those for medical care?

Yes	1*
No	2

Dept. of Health clinic	Union health center
Chest clinic	Settlement house
Well-baby clinic	H.I.P. health center
Welfare eye clinic	Cancer detection clinic
Catholic Charities	Aftercare clinic
Protestant welfare agencies	Mental health clinic
Jewish family service	Child guidance clinic

*IF YES: Which one? Any others? (*Record EXACT NAME AND ADDRESS below, or else record most accurate possible description and location of clinic*)

6. IF YES TO EITHER Q. 4 OR Q. 5, ASK BOTH "A" & "B" SEPARATELY FOR EACH CLINIC LISTED BELOW:

A. How many times did (you, name) go to (clinic)? (*Record below*)

B. How many of those times did you actually see a doctor? (*Record below*)

NAME:_____

OTHER CLINICS (NON-HOSPITAL)

Name of Clinic	Address	Total Number of Visits	No. Times Doctor Seen

7. Since (date of first interview), did (you, name) see any of these kinds of doctors *in your home or in his private office*? (HAND REVERSE SIDE OF BLUE CARD)

Yes	1*
No	2

Welfare doctor   Camp doctor
Compensation doctor   Insurance doctor
School doctor   H.I.P. doctor
Employment doctor   Private doctor

*A. IF YES: Which? Any other kinds of doctors there that (you, name) saw at home or in his private office since (date)? (*Record TYPE OF DOCTOR in space below*)

ASK "B" & "C" FOR EACH TYPE NAMED AND RECORD BELOW. IF NONE, ENTER ZERO.

B. How many visits did the (type of doctor) make to your home?

C. How many visits did you make to the (type of doctor's) office?

Type of dr.

No. visits _____ home _____home _____ home _____ home _____home

No. visits _____ office_____office_____ office _____ office _____ office

NAME:_____

8. Since (date of last interview), did (you, name) go to any *dentist*? (or school dental clinic?

	Yes	1*
	No	2

*IF YES, ASK BOTH "A" & "B"

A. Was this in a dental clinic?

	Yes	1*
	No	2

*IF YES, ASK:

(1) What clinic was that?_____

(2) Any others? _____

(3) How many times altogether did (you, name) see a dentist at any clinic? _____

B. Did (you, name) go to any private dentist?

	Yes	1*
	No	2

*IF YES, ASK:

(1) How many times did (you, name) see a private dentist? _____

NOW FILL OUT UTILIZATION SUPPLEMENT FOR NEXT CASE MEMBER.

WHEN UTILIZATION SUPPLEMENTS HAVE BEEN COMPLETED FOR ALL CASE MEMBERS, RETURN TO QUESTION 2 ON MAIN QUESTIONNAIRE.

CONFIDENTIAL
Survey 478
7-63

ENTER CASE NO.

NATIONAL OPINION RESEARCH CENTER
University of Chicago

H E A L T H   C A R E   S T U D Y

THIRD WAVE

ASK ONLY IF PRESENT ADDRESS IS DIFFERENT FROM
2nd WAVE INTERVIEW:

A. First tell me, how long have you been
   living at this address? _____

                                              months

   (1) Where were you living before that? _____

   (2) And how long had you been living there? _____
                                       (Specify years, months or days)

B. Now I need a list of all the people who live in this household. (LIST RESPOND-
   ENT ON FIRST LINE.) Besides yourself, who else lives here? Let's take them in
   order of age. (CONTINUE LISTING ALL HOUSEHOLD MEMBERS.)

C. Have we missed any children or babies or anyone else who lives here -- anyone
   away travelling, in a hospital, visiting somewhere, or in an institution? (IF YES,
   ADD TO LISTING)

DRAW A LINE UNDER LAST NAME LISTED AND THEN ASK "D"

D. Has anyone else lived in this household since (date of 2nd wave interview), who
   isn't living here now? (IF YES, ADD NAME TO LISTING)

E. FOR EACH PERSON LISTED, RECORD RELATIONSHIP TO RESPONDENT,
   AGE, SEX, MARITAL STATUS (M-S-W-D-Sep) AND NUMBER OF MONTHS
   IN HOUSEHOLD SINCE 2nd WAVE INTERVIEW.

Last Name	First Name	Relation to Resp.	Age	Sex	Marital Status	No. of Months

HAVE ALL CASE MEMBERS LISTED ON YELLOW FACE SHEET BEEN
LISTED ABOVE? IF NOT, RECORD PRESENT ADDRESS ON EACH ABSENT
CASE MEMBER ON FACE SHEET.

HAVE ANY NEW BABIES BEEN BORN TO A MOTHER IN THE CASE SINCE
SECOND WAVE INTERVIEW? IF YES, ADD THE CHILD TO THE LIST OF
CASE MEMBERS ON YELLOW FACE SHEET.

1. A. Would you say your own health, in general, is excellent, good, fair, or poor?

   B. IF SPOUSE IN CASE: How about the health of your (spouse) – In general, would you rate it as excellent, good, fair, or poor?

   C. IF CHILDREN IN CASE: How about the health of the child(ren), in general?

	A Self	B Spouse	C Children
Excellent	8-1	9-1	10-1
Good	2	2	2
Fair	3	3	3
Poor	4	4	4
Don't know	5	5	5

REFER TO BACK OF THIRD WAVE FACE SHEET AND RECORD UNDER Q. 2 AND AGAIN UNDER Q. 3 THE NUMBERS AND NAMES, *IN NUMERICAL ORDER*, OF ALL CONDITIONS RESPONDENT HAD TWO YEARS AGO. USE YOUR "INTERVIEWER'S ILLNESS GUIDE" FOR NAMES OF CONDITIONS.

IF NO CONDITIONS LISTED ON FACE SHEET, CHECK BOX AND SKIP TO Q. 4 ON PAGE 4.

2. A. Have you had (1st condition) at any time during the past *two* years? – that is, since the very first time we talked with you.

   IF DON'T KNOW, PROBE: Did a doctor tell you you had (condition) at any time during the last two years?

   CODE UNDER "A" ON OPPOSITE PAGE

   IF NO OR DON'T KNOW, GO ON TO NEXT CONDITION

   *IF YES, ASK BOTH "B" & "C"

   B. Do you have (condition) now?

   ALTERNATE WORDING: Have you recently had (condition)?

   C. During the past two years, did you see a doctor about your (condition)?

REPEAT FOR EACH CONDITION LISTED, THEN GO BACK TO Q. 3.

3. Two years ago, when we first talked with you, you mentioned that you had (1st condition listed). *ASK EITHER "A" OR "B"*

    A. IF "YES" TO Q. 2-B: I see now that you still have (condition). In general, would you say it has remained the same, improved, or become worse during the past two years? (*Record verbatim*)

    B. IF "NO" TO Q. 2-B: I see now that you don't have (condition) any more. Can you tell me about that? (*Record verbatim*)

2. CONDITIONS RESPONDENT HAD TWO YEARS AGO

		A Has had during past two years			B Has now		C Saw Doctor	
No.	Name of Condition	Yes	No	DK	Yes	No	Yes	No
		R*	1	2	3	4	W	Z
		R*	1	2	3	4	W	Z
		R*	1	2	3	4	W	Z
		R*	1	2	3	4	W	Z
		R*	1	2	3	4	W	Z
		R*	1	2	3	4	W	Z
		R*	1	2	3	4	W	Z
		R*	1	2	3	4	W	Z
		R*	1	2	3	4	W	Z
					79-5		80-0	

3. CONDITIONS RESPONDENT HAD TWO YEARS AGO

No.	Name of Condition	Verbatim Answer to "A" or "B"	1-6

4. What (other) illnesses, or injuries, have you had during the past two years? (LIST BELOW, THEN PROBE: Any others?)

None   1

FOR EACH ONE LISTED, ASK "A" AND CODE YES OR NO

A. Did you see a doctor about (condition)?

OTHER ILLNESSES OR INJURIES DURING PAST TWO YEARS	A Saw Doctor	
	Yes	No
	1	2
	1	2
	1	2
	1	2
	1	2
	79-5	80-1

NOW MAKE OUT A UTILIZATION SUPPLEMENT FOR EACH CASE MEMBER, INCLUDING ANY NEW BABIES ADDED TO LIST ON BACK OF SECOND WAVE FACE SHEET AND INCLUDING ANY CASE MEMBERS DECEASED SINCE THE SECOND WAVE INTERVIEW.

1-6

IF NO MEDICAL CARE THIS YEAR,
CHECK BOX AND SKIP TO Q. 6. ☐

FROM THIRD WAVE FACE SHEET AND FROM EACH UTILIZATION SUP-PLEMENT, LIST BELOW EACH DIFFERENT *HOSPITAL*, *NON-HOSPITAL CLINIC* AND *TYPE OF DOCTOR* USED DURING LAST *TWO* YEARS

Hospitals _____

Non-Hospital Clinics _____

Type of doctors (include
only HIP, Welfare, Private
doctors and private
psychiatrists from Q. 6 of
Supplements) _____

IF NONE OR ONLY ONE PLACE LISTED ON THREE LINES ABOVE, ☐
CHECK BOX AND SKIP TO Q. 6.

IF TWO OR MORE PLACES LISTED ABOVE, ASK Q. 5.

5. Some people (families) use only one place for all their medical care, while others use more than one. I see that you (your family) have used (*name all places listed on lines above*) during the last two years.

How is it that you did not get all your medical care in one place?

7-

8-

9-

10-

---

6. (Even though you have not had any medical care these past two years) Do you think of any one place as the *main* place to get your (family's) medical care?

Yes	11-1*
No (SKIP TO Q. 7)	2

*IF YES, ASK BOTH "A" & "B"

A. What place is that?

12-
13-

B. If you should need any medical care during the next year, would there be any circumstances at all under which you would use some other place?

Yes	14-1**
No (SKIP TO Q. 8)	2
Don't know (SKIP TO Q. 8)	3

**IF YES TO "B", ASK BOTH "C" & "D"

15-
16-

C. Where else might you go? (Any other place?)

17-
18-
19-

D. Under what circumstances are you likely to use (*each place named in "C"*)?

20-

21-
22-
23-
24-

NOW SKIP TO Q. 8.

ASK Q. 7 ONLY IF "NO" TO Q. 6

7. A. If you should need medical care next year, which place or places do you think you would probably use?

IF DON'T KNOW OR NONE, SKIP TO Q. 8

B. Are you likely to use any other places? (IF YES) Which? (Any place else?)

IF MORE THAN ONE MENTIONED IN "A" AND "B", ASK "C"

C. Under what circumstances are you likely to use (*each place listed in A or B*)?

---

8. ASK EVERYONE: In general, do you think it's a good idea to try to get *all* of your medical care in one place, or is it better to go to different places depending on the circumstances?

One place	25-1
Different places	2
Don't know	3
	26-

---

9. Now a question about different illness conditions. Suppose a person had "arthritis or rheumatism." Do you think a doctor could cure it completely, could he help it but perhaps not cure it, or couldn't he help it at all? How about (*continue with list, repeating question as necessary*)?

	Complete Cure	Help Not Cure	Couldn't Help	Don't Know	DK Illness
1. Arthritis or rheumatism	27-1	2	3	4	5
2. Heart trouble	28-1	2	3	4	5
3. Tonsillitis	29-1	2	3	4	5
4. Diabetes	30-1	2	3	4	5
5. Gall bladder trouble	31-1	2	3	4	5
6. Tuberculosis	32-1	2	3	4	5
7. Cancer	33-1	2	3	4	5

---

10. What do you think *causes* (*each illness below*)? – just your own ideas of what causes it?

A. Heart trouble:
       34-
       35-
       36-
       37-

B. Tuberculosis:
       38-
       39-
       40-
       41-

C. Diabetes: 42-
                                                                    43-
                                                                    44-
                                                                    45-

D. Cancer   46-
                                                                    47-
                                                                    48-
                                                                    49-

50-   51-

IF NO MEDICAL CARE DURING PAST YEAR, SKIP TO Q. 12.

11. Altogether, would you say the medical care you (your family) got this past year was better, about the same, or worse than the medical care you got the year before?

Better	52-1*
About the same	2
Worse	3*
Don't know	4

*A. IF BETTER OR WORSE: In what way was it (better/worse)?

53-

54-

12. If you could choose, and it didn't cost you anything, would you rather go to a *hospital* clinic or emergency room, or would you rather see a private doctor?

Clinic or emergency room	55-1
Private doctor	2
Don't know	3

13. Is there any *one* person you think of as your own doctor?

Yes	56-1
No	2
Don't know	3

14. When you go to a clinic, how important is it that you see the same doctor each time -- is it very important to you, fairly important, or not important at all?

Very important	57-1*
Fairly important	2*
Not important	3
Don't know	4

*A. IF VERY OR FAIRLY IMPORTANT: Do you *usually* get to see the same
doctor each time you go to the clinic?

Yes	58-1
No	2
Qualified (*specify*)	3
Don't know	4

---

15. Here are some things people sometimes say about doctors. I'd like to know
whether you personally think they are true (of your own doctor) (doctors you
yourself have seen) or not? For example, (READ "A"). Do you think that is
true of (your own doctor) (doctors you have seen) or not? (*Continue through
list, circling one code for each.*)

	True of Own Dr.	Not True	Don't Know
A. Your doctor(s) doesn't (don't) give you a chance to tell him (them) exactly what your trouble is	59-1	2	3
B. Your doctor doesn't take enough personal interest in you	60-1	2	3
C. Your doctor wants you to come back for additional visits even if you don't need them	61-1	2	3
D. Your doctor doesn't tell you enough about your condition; he doesn't explain just what the trouble is	62-1	2	3
E. Your doctor gives better care to his private patients than to his clinic patients	63-1	2	3
F. Your doctor tells you there is nothing wrong with you when you know there is	64-1	2	3
G. Your doctor rushes too much when he examines you	65-1	2	3
H. Your doctor is a very understanding person	66-1	2	3
I. Your doctor goes out of his way to help you	67-1	2	3

---

16. Now I'll read the list again and I'd like you to tell me whether you think each
one is true of *most* doctors, or not. (*Repeat, circling one code for each.*)

	True of Most Drs.	Not True	Don't Know
A. Most doctors don't give their patients a chance to to tell them exactly what their trouble is	68-1	2	3
B. Most doctors don't take enough personal interest in their patients	69-1	2	3
C. Most doctors want their patients to come back for additional visits even if they don't need them	70-1	2	3
D. Most doctors don't tell their patients enough about their condition; they don't explain just what the trouble is	71-1	2	3
E. Most doctors give better care to their private patients than to their clinic patients	72-1	2	3
F. Most doctors tell their patients there's nothing wrong with him when he knows there is	73-1	2	3

	True of Most Drs.	Not True	Don't Know
G. Most doctors rush too much when they examine their patients	74-1	2	3
H. Most doctors are understanding people	75-1	2	3
I. Most doctors go out of their way to help the patient	76-1	2	3
77-	78-	79-5	80-2

17. Now here are some things people say about *hospitals*. When I say each one, I want you to tell me *which* hospital or hospitals in New York City seem that way to you. It doesn't matter if you haven't been there yourself -- you may have heard other people talk about them.

Now which hospital seems to you *easy to get to*? (*CONTINUE THROUGH LIST, WRITING IN ALL COMMENTS VERBATIM*)

A. Easy to get to?

7-
8-
9-
10-

B. Good, but too far away?

11-
12-
13-
14-

C. Has the best doctors?

15-
16-
17-
18-

D. Keeps you waiting much too long?

19-
20-
21-
22-

E. Only for rich people?

23-
24-
25-
26-

F. Overcrowded?

27-
28-
29-
30-

G. Not enough doctors and nurses?

31-
32-
33-
34-

H. Friendly?

35-
36-
37-
38-

I. Gloomy, or dirty?

39-
40-
41-
42-

J. Doesn't treat you like a person?

43-
44-
45-
46-

REFER TO UPPER RIGHT CORNER OF YELLOW FACE SHEET.

IF RESPONDENT IS PART OF NYH PROJECT ("A" OR "B"), ASK Q. 18.

IF RESPONDENT IS NOT PART OF PROJECT ("C"). SKIP TO Q. 24 ON P. 12.

---

18. A. Did you (your family) receive a letter asking you to go to the New York Hospital for all your medical care?

Yes	47-1
No	2*
Don't know	3*

*B. IF NO OR DK: Have you ever heard of the New York Hospital Project?

Yes	48-1
No	2

REFER TO BOX ON PAGE 5.

IF N. Y. HOSPITAL LISTED THERE, GO ON TO Q. 20.

IF N. Y. HOSPITAL *NOT* LISTED AND *"YES"* TO *EITHER* Q. 18-A or B, ASK Qs. 19 & 20, THEN SKIP TO Q. 24.

IF N. Y. HOSPITAL *NOT* LISTED AND *"NO"* OR "DK" TO *BOTH* Qs. 18-A & B, SKIP DIRECTLY TO Q. 24.

---

19. I see you didn't use the New York Hospital this year or last year. Why is it that you did not go there at all? (Any other reasons?)

49-
50-
51-
52-

---

20. As far as you know, which of these services could you get at the New York Hospital if you needed them -- For example (*read each item and code under Q. 20*)

IF RESPONDENT VOLUNTEERS THAT HE
USED ANY SERVICES, CIRCLE UNDER
Q. 21.

	Q. 20 Yes No DK	Q. 21- Used
A. Would a doctor from the New York Hospital come to your home if you needed him?	53-1 2 3	Z
B. Would a nurse from the New York Hospital make home visits	54-1 2 3	Z
C. Could you get psychiatric care if you needed it?	55-1 2 3	Z

	Q. 20			Q. 21-
	Yes	No	DK	Used
D. Could you get medical advice by telephone during the day?	56-1	2	3	Z
E. Could you get medical advice by telephone at night or on weekends?	57-1	2	3	Z
F. Would they pay your carfare to get to the clinic?	58-1	2	3	Z
G. If you were very sick, would they get an ambulance or taxi to take you to New York Hospital?	59-1	2	3	Z
H. Are there any medical services you could *not* get from New York Hospital if you needed them?	60-1	2	3	Z
(IF YES) Which? Any others?	61-			
	62-			None Z
	63-			
	64-			

IF N. Y. HOSPITAL *NOT* LISTED IN BOX ON P. 5, SKIP TO Q. 24.
Qs. 21-23 ARE ASKED ONLY OF THOSE WHO HAVE USED N. Y. HOSPITAL IN LAST TWO YEARS.

---

21. HAND RESPONDENT WHITE CARD. Here is a list of those services I just asked you about.

    Did you (your family) use (any of them at N.Y. Hospital) (any others besides the ones you mentioned) during the last two years? (IF YES) Which ones? Any others? (*Code under Q. 21 above*)

---

22. What were some of the things you liked best about the New York Hospital? (Could you explain and tell me a little more about that?)

65-

66-

67-

68-

69-

70-

71-

72-

23. And what were some of the things you did not like so much about the New York Hospital? (Even though you liked it, we're interested in any little things you may not have been too satisfied with.)

73-

74-

75-

76-

77-

78-

79-5

80-3

1-6

ASK EVERYBODY:

24. Up to now we have been asking questions about your health. Now I have a few different questions.   7-

A. How long have you been living in New York City?

Less than 3 years	8-1*
3-4 years	2*
5-9 years	3*
10-14 years	4*
15-19 years	5*
20 years or more	6
All my life	7

OMIT "B" IF 20 YEARS OR MORE OR "ALL MY LIFE"

*B. Before you came to live in New York City, were you living in a small village, a town or a big city?

Small village	9-1
Town	2
Big city	3
Other (*specify*)	4

25. What was your father's main occupation when you were about 16?

10-
11-

26. A. What was the most skilled job that you yourself ever had? (IF VAGUE, PROBE: What actually did you do on that job?)

                                                 12-

     Occupation: _____   13-

     Industry: _____

   B. And about when was that?
     (*Probe for approximate years.*)   _____   14-

---

27. A. IF RESPONDENT FEMALE AND HUSBAND IN CASE: What was the most skilled job your husband ever had? (IF VAGUE, PROBE: What did he actually do on that job?)

                                                 15-

     Occupation: _____   16-

     Industry: _____

   B. And about when was that?
     (*Probe for approximate years.*)   _____   17-

---

28. Finally I have some questions about welfare or public assistance. I'll read you some things people sometimes say about Welfare, and I'd like to know for each one whether you *agree with it* or *disagree with it*. The first one is . . .

	Agree	Disagree	Don't Know
A. Welfare refuses assistance to many people when they really need it	18-1	2	3
B. Most people would not apply for Welfare if they could possibly manage without it	19-1	2	3
C. Welfare investigators give people a hard time when they don't have to	20-1	2	3
D. Lots of people on Welfare are chiselers -- they get money from Welfare that they're not entitled to	21-1	2	3
E. If you treat people on Welfare too well, no one will want to work	22-1	2	3
F. People who apply for Welfare are made to feel humiliated	23-1	2	3
G. Welfare just doesn't give people enough money to live on	24-1	2	3
H. Welfare interferes too much in your private life	25-1	2	3

---

29. Out of every hundred people in New York City right now, about how many would you think receive money from Welfare -- Would you guess about 1 person out of every hundred is on Welfare, or about 5 in a hundred, or 10, or what? (Just your best guess)

30. Have you yourself ever received money from Welfare?

Yes	27-R*
No (SKIP TO Q. 36)	1

*A. IF YES: Do you receive any money from Welfare now?

Yes	2
No (SKIP TO Q. 32)	3

---

31. Since you were first on Welfare, was there any period of time when you were off?

Yes	28-1
No (SKIP TO Q. 33)	2

---

32. When you went off Welfare (the last time), was this all right with you or did you feel that you should have been kept on?

All right	29-1
Kept on	2*
Don't know	3*

*A. IF KEPT ON OR DON'T KNOW: Why do you feel that way?

30-

31-

---

33. Does being on or off Welfare make any difference at all in the *medical care* you can get?

Yes	32-1*
No	2
Don't know	3

*A. IF YES: In what way?

33-

34-

35-

36-

34. ASK ONLY IF RESPONDENT IS PART OF NYH PROJECT AND YES TO Q. 30

As far as you know, could you get medical care at the New York Hospital Project during these past two years, even during periods when you might be off Welfare?

Yes	37-1
No	2
Don't know	3

35. Are there any other things you would like to say about Welfare and Welfare investigators?

38-

39-

40-

41-

42-

43-

36. IF SPOUSE IN CASE: How many years of school did your (spouse) finish?

Never attended school	44-1	Completed 8 years	5
Completed 1-3 years	2	Completed 9-11 years	6
Completed 4-5 years	3	Completed 12 years	7
Completed 6-7 years	4	More than 12 years	8

37. ASK ALL NON-PROJECT RESPONDENTS

Have you ever heard of the New York Hospital Project?

Yes	45-1*
No	2
Don't know	3

*IF YES, ASK BOTH "A" & "B"

A. How did you hear about it?

B. What did you hear about it?

46-

47-

48-

49-

A. How long did this interview take?

B. RESPONDENT'S ATTITUDE
   WAS: (*Circle one*):

Friendly, eager	50-1
Cooperative	2
Passive, indifferent	3
Hostile, suspicious	4

C. Was any other person present
   while you were conducting
   the interview?

Yes	51-R*
No	1

*IF YES: Do you think this
affected his answers in any way?
(*If Yes, explain*)

D. Was communication with
   this respondent difficult
   for any reason (besides
   language)?

Yes (Explain)	52-R
No	1

E. INTERVIEWER'S
   SIGNATURE: 53-
                              54-

F. DATE OF INTERVIEW: 55-
                          56-
                          57-

AFTER CHECKING THIS
INTERVIEW FOR RECORDING
ERRORS OR OMISSIONS,
ATTACH FACE SHEETS TO
FIRST PAGE.

NORC: 478   3rd Wave

HEALTH CARE STUDY

UTILIZATION SUPPLEMENT

NAME:_____   CASE NO._____

Up to now we have been talking about the last two years. Now I want to ask you some questions about any medical and dental care that (you or name of case member) have had since the last time we talked with you about a year ago on (date of 2nd wave interview)

1. First, since (date of 2nd wave interview) did (you, name) go to any dentist (or school dental clinic)?

Yes	1*
No	2

*IF YES, ASK BOTH A & B

    A. Was this a dental clinic?

Yes	1**
No	2

    **IF YES TO "A", ASK (1) & (2)

        (1) What clinic was that?_____
                        (Record name and location)

        IF HOSPITAL DENTAL CLINIC, RECORD UNDER Q. 2 BELOW

        (2) Any others?

    B. Did (you, name) go to any private dentist?

Yes	1#
No	2

    #(1) IF YES TO "B": How many times did (you, name) see a private dentist since (date of 2nd wave interview)?

---

2. Did (you, name) have to stay overnight or longer in any hospital or mental institution since (date of 2nd wave)?

Yes	1*
No	2

*IF YES, ASK A-B-C-D

    A. What hospital was that? (*Record at bottom of page*)
    B. How many different *times* were (you, name) a bed patient in that hospital since (date)? (*Record name of hospital on SEPARATE LINE FOR EACH ADMISSION*)

NAME:_____

C. What condition were (you, name) in the hospital for (that time)? (*Record for each admission*)

D. Did (you, name) have to stay overnight in any other hospital or mental institution since (date)?

IF NO, GO ON TO Q. 3.

IF YES, REPEAT A, B, C & D

HOSPITAL	CONDITION FOR WHICH HOSPITALIZED

3. Since (date of 2nd wave interview) did (you, name) go to any *hospital clinic or emergency room*?

Yes	1*
No	2

*IF YES, ASK FOLLOWING SERIES

A. At what hospital was that? (*Record below*)

B. Did you go to the clinic or to the emergency room?

IF CLINIC: *Probe for exact name of clinic and record below.*

IF EMERGENCY ROOM: *Record "Emerg." below.*

IF BOTH: *Use two lines below.*

C. Since (date), did (you, name) go to any other hospital clinic or emergency room?

IF NO, GO ON TO "D" & "E"

IF YES, RECORD HOSPITAL NAME BELOW, THEN REPEAT "B" & "C"

NOW ASK "D" & "E" SEPARATELY FOR EACH LINE BELOW

D. About how many times did (you, name) go to (name of clinic or emergency room) since (date of last interview)? (*Record below*)

E. And how many of those times did (you, name) actually see a doctor? (*Record below*)

NAME:_____

4. Since (date of 2nd wave interview) did a Home Care doctor *from a hospital clinic* come to see (you, name) at your home?

Yes	1*
No	2

*IF YES, RECORD "HOME CARE" UNDER "B" BELOW AND ASK (1), (2), (3)

(1) From what hospital did he come? (*Record under "A" below*)

(2) How many times did he visit (you, name)? (Record under "D" below)

(3) Did a Home Care doctor from any other hospital clinic come to see (you, name) since (date of 2nd wave interview)?

IF YES, WRITE "HOME CARE" ON NEW LINE UNDER "B" AND REPEAT (1) - (3)

HOSPITAL CLINICS OR EMERGENCY ROOMS

A. Hospital	B. Name of Clinic or Emergency Room	D. Total Number of Visits	E. No. Times Doctor Seen

5. Since (date of 2nd wave interview), did (you, name) go to any of these kinds of *non-hospital* clinics or health centers? (*HAND RESPONDENT YELLOW CARD*)

Yes	1*
No	2

Dept. of Health clinic	Union Health center	Protestant Welfare Agencies
Chest clinic	Settlement house	Jewish Family Service
Welfare eye clinic	HIP health center	After care clinic
Catholic Charities	Cancer detection clinic	Well-baby clinic (including
Child Guidance Clinic	Mental health clinic	those in either Bellevue or
		Metropolitan Hospitals)

*IF YES, ASK BOTH "A" & "B"

A. Which one? Any others? (*Record EXACT NAME AND ADDRESS below, of each clinic mentioned, or else record most accurate possible description and location*)

B. Since (date of 2nd wave interview), did you go to any other non-hospital clinics which are not listed on the card? (IF YES, REPEAT "A")

NAME:_____

FOR EACH CLINIC RECORDED BELOW, ASK "C" & "D"

C. How many times did (you, name) go to (clinic)? (*Record under C below*)

D. And how many times did you actually see a doctor? (*Record under D below*)

OTHER CLINICS (NON-HOSPITAL)

Name of Clinic	Address	C Total Number of Visits	D No. Times Doctor Seen

6. Since (date of 2nd wave interview), did (you, name) see any of these kinds of doctors *either in your home or in his private office*?

	Yes	1*
	No	2

Welfare doctor	Employment doctor	HIP doctor
Compensation doctor	Camp doctor	Private doctor
School doctor	Insurance doctor	Private psychiatrist

*A. IF YES: Which? Any other kinds of doctors there that (you, name) saw at home or in his private office since (date)? (*Record TYPE OF DOCTOR in space below*)

ASK "B" & "C" FOR EACH TYPE NAMED AND RECORD BELOW. IF NONE, ENTER ZERO.

B. How many visits did the (type of doctor) make to your home?

C. How many visits did you make to the (type of doctor's) office?

Type of dr.
_____

No. visits _____home ____home ____home ____home ____home

No. visits _____office ____office ____office ____office ____office

ASK Q. 7 ONLY IF FEMALE 14-50 YEARS OLD. OTHERWISE FOLLOW IN-STRUCTIONS AT BOTTOM.

7. (Have you) (Has name) been pregnant at any time during the last *two* years?

Yes	1*
No	2

IF NO, GO ON TO NEXT SUPPLEMENT OR RETURN TO MAIN QUESTIONNAIRE

*A. IF YES: How many times (were you) (was name) pregnant during the last two years?

Once	1
Twice	2
Three times	3

B. FOR EACH PREGNANCY, ASK: In what kind of place was the baby born – that is, was he born in a hospital, or at home, or somewhere else? (*CODE BELOW. If "Somewhere else", specify. If not a live birth, specify under "Other result"*)

IF PRIVATE DOCTOR SEEN THIS YEAR (Q. 6-U) OR LAST YEAR (WHITE FACE SHEET), ASK "C"

C. Did (you, name) see a private doctor during the (first) pregnancy, before the baby was born? (*Code below*)

IF YES, ASK BOTH "D" & "E"

D. During which month of (your, name's) pregnancy did (you, name) first see a doctor? (*Record below*)

E. And how many times did (you, name) see a doctor for the (first) pregnancy? (*Record below*)

REPEAT "C" FOR SECOND AND THIRD PREGNANCIES, IF ANY

	First pregnancy		Second pregnancy		Third pregnancy	
B. RESULT OF PREGNANCY	Live birth:		Live birth:		Live birth:	
	Hospital	1	Hospital	1	Hospital	1
	Home	2	Home	2	Home	2
	Other place	3	Other place	3	Other place	3
	Other result:		Other result:		Other result:	
C. SAW DOCTOR?	Yes	1	Yes	1	Yes	1
	No	2	No	2	No	2
	Don't know	3	Don't know	3	Don't know	3

D. MONTH FIRST
   SAW DOCTOR:

E. NO. TIMES
   SAW DOCTOR:

NOW FILL OUT UTILIZATION SUPPLEMENT FOR NEXT CASE MEMBER.

WHEN UTILIZATION SUPPLEMENTS HAVE BEEN COMPLETED FOR ALL CASE MEMBERS, RETURN TO PAGE 5 ON MAIN QUESTIONNAIRE.

Appendix C

Clinical and Research Definitions of Adults and Children

Comparisons between the study and control groups have been made in terms of defined population sub-groups (children under 13 at intake, teenagers then 13–17, adults in multi-person welfare cases, and so on). Because the Project population was randomly drawn from a section of the community – new admissions to welfare in the local district – the generalization of its conclusions (with the usual cautions) requires precise definitions of the various sub-groups.

However, when the 1,204 people in the study group who responded to the invitation entered the New York Hospital, they were viewed not as representatives of specific sub-groups in the community but simply as patients. The way in which clinicians classify patients does not necessarily coincide with the statistician's neat groupings: for instance, the first division in an out-patient department is between adults to be seen in the medical (and surgical, obstetrical, and other) clinics and the children to be seen in pediatrics. Children at the New York Hospital are usually seen in pediatrics until the age of 13 or 14 and then transferred to medicine; but the dividing line is not a rigid one. The size or maturity of the child, or the point in time at which he first comes for medical care, may be taken into consideration.

After much discussion, it was decided that in Chapters 6 through 8 the Project patients would be classified as adults (that is, patients seen by internists) and children (that is, patients seen by pediatricians) because that was how they were actually cared for on the Project; but in other chapters, reporting the experimental findings, the divisions would be into rigidly defined sub-groups in the population. The chief discrepancy lies with the teenagers, who were seen either in pediatrics or medicine and sometimes consecutively in both. The following tabulation bridges the gap between the two terminologies, and shows the relationship of the medical and pediatric clinic loads to the welfare terminology employed elsewhere.

Medical patients

Single adults	376
Family adults	260
Teenagers	48
Total	684

Pediatric patients

Children originally invited	469
New babies	51
Total	520
Total Patients	1,204

Appendix D

Methods of Record-Checking

The home interviews were chiefly relied on for identifying the sources of care patients had used during the two year experimental period. They proved better as sources of actual utilization rates than anticipated, and the records were less adequate than expected. This fact was established by a check of reported versus recorded information in a subsample of the cases.

Ambulant Care

In the home interviews, 12 months and 24 months after intake respectively, respondents were asked if they or any other members of their welfare case had visited a clinic in a hospital. If the answer was affirmative, they were asked to specify the hospital, the clinic or emergency room within the hospital and the number of visits to each.

A thorough record check was instituted for every person in the two subsamples – 100 study group cases and 100 control group cases. The study group subsample contained 253 persons, 13 of them babies born during the Project. The control group subsample contained 271 persons, 24 of them new babies.

The name of every person in the subsamples was checked through the index of in-patients and out-patients in the following hospitals, whether or not he reported using it: New York Hospital; Bellevue; Metropolitan; Mount Sinai. (There was sometimes one index for all patients, for example, at New York Hospital and Mount Sinai, and sometimes one or more different files for in-patients, separate from the out-patient index, for example, at Metropolitan. Bellevue had six separate indexes.) In addition, the name was checked through the index of other hospitals if: the person himself reported going there during the study period; the person himself reported going there within five years before intake; another case member reported going there during the study period.

The results of the record check were recorded as follows: (1) If out-patient visits were found, record was made of names of clinics, dates, number of visits, number of different doctors seen, and condition or diagnosis if noted. (2) If no out-patient visits were found, a distinction was drawn between the following reasons for this: medical chart found and no visits entered within the study period; name indexed but no chart found; name not indexed. Hospitals not indexed included those which refused permission and those in outlying parts of the city with only one or two patients reporting utilization there.

An attempt was made to check the names of all the children in the subsamples for non-hospital clinic visits through the records of the child health stations in the areas in which they lived; but when, after an intensive effort, only one third of the records had been located, this attempt was abandoned.

No checking of private doctor or welfare panel physician records was attempted. The latter was theoretically possible but the expected yield did not appear to justify the work involved. (Welfare panel physician visits are entered on punch cards by the Welfare Department for accounting purposes; but when the monthly accounts have been summarized, the individual IBM cards are destroyed.)

Careful analysis was then made of the extent of correspondence between reported and recorded hospital utilization in the 253 study group persons and the 271 control group persons. Hospital records, it turned out, varied greatly in their adequacy. The records at the New York Hospital were excellent and so was the patient index through which one could trace whether or not a particular patient had a record at the hospital. But the hospitals used most by the control group (and by many of the study group too) were the two local city hospitals, Bellevue and Metropolitan, and here the situation was very different. These are both very large hospitals, with a turnover of many hundreds of thousands of different patients, including many Puerto Ricans, whose similarity of names and frequency of changing them makes them especially difficult to trace through a patient index. It proved hard to make a positive identification in some instances, despite the availability from Project records of present and past addresses, family constellation, and names of parents. (Names of parents, especially mother's maiden name, proved the most useful piece of identifying information one could have on a patient.) Even when the patient's name was identified, the record often could not be found or was incomplete; this was particularly likely to happen at Bellevue.

Reported visits, on the other hand, turned out to be surprisingly accurate in the aggregate. Individual patients over- and under-reported, often considerably, so that estimates for small groups of patients are unreliable; but the over- and under-reporting tended to balance, so that for relatively large numbers of patients, the interviews appear to yield reasonably reliable estimates. Because of the unevenness of the other hospital records, the New York Hospital records were used as the criterion for the "real" number of visits that took place. When visits to the New York Hospital reported by or on behalf of the 511 patients in the subsamples were compared with those found in the record, a ratio of approximately 0.9 was obtained, that is, for every 10 visits reported, 9 were found in the record. (It may be remembered that utilization questions covered all case members but that the information could be obtained from any member of the household or, indeed, from any person who seemed qualified to answer.)

A 100 per cent record check at the New York Hospital was eventually completed on all persons in the study and control group, whether or not they reported using the New York Hospital, so that reported versus recorded visits could be compared for the whole population. Slightly more over-reporting occurred for the whole group than for the subsample, but the difference was not great: it was about 12 per cent instead of 10 per cent. It was therefore decided that, rather than go through the complexities of developing a "correction factor" for the over- and under-reporters (a factor that would vary from one sub-group to another), the number of ambulant visits would be accepted as reported to NORC by those who were interviewed. The 10 to 12 per cent over-reporting, in any case, was roughly balanced by the visits made by those not interviewed.

Acute In-patient Admissions

In the last two home interviews respondents were asked if they or any other members of the case had been a bed patient in a hospital during the year. If the answer was "yes," they were asked the name of the hospital and the number of times they had been admitted there. They were not specifically asked the number of days they stayed because it had been found in a pre-test that estimates of length of stay were very inaccurate. However, many respondents volunteered information about reason for hospitalization, dates and length of stay; all such remarks were recorded verbatim by the NORC interviewers.

Because an in-patient admission is a much larger item of medical cost than an out-patient visit and because more in-patient utilization than out-patient utilization might be lost from failure to interview (sicker patients might die or remain in institutions), every effort was made to secure records on in-patient admissions.

There were six sources of information leading to in-patient data: (1) All reported hospitalizations were investigated. (2) When a patient reported one hospitalization during the study period and his chart was found, it was searched for possible readmissions during the study. (3) References within one hospital chart to admissions to another institution were followed up. (4) All patients in the two sub-samples were checked through the major hospitals and other likely ones for in-patient admissions as described under the procedure for out-patient care. (5) All patients who died were checked through the four main hospitals as well as any others their records suggested they might have used. (6) Hospitalizations were counted (whether or not the actual record was located) for the mothers of all babies born during the study, unless the interview stated the birth occurred outside a hospital. (When the record was not found, four days were allowed for in-patient admission.)

In-patient records are thus not guaranteed to be absolutely complete, but it is felt that few were missed after this rather exhaustive search. As a check, an investigation was made of the New York Hospital admissions (believed to be 100 per cent complete as a result of complete indexing of all patients) to see how many would have been missed without this indexing, that is, using the same methods as were used at the other hospitals. Ten admissions the first year and 11 the second, out of a total of 354 admissions, belonged in this category; they were nearly all very brief admissions, several being overnight only.

Chronic Institutional Care

As noted in Chapter 10, the admissions to chronic institutions were the hardest to document, mostly because the interviews were least helpful here. All possible clues to long-term institutionalization were followed up, and where definitive records could not be found, a best estimate of the incidence of hospitalization, and of length of stay, was made individually for each case by a group of the research staff.

Appendix E

Source of Unit Costs

Voluntary Hospitals

In-patient Services: per diem costs. The 1962 costs were based on the expenditures of 53 United Hospital Fund members, all general hospitals. These are divided into four categories: hospitals with obstetrical service, with school of nursing (24); hospitals with obstetrical service, without school of nursing (17); hospitals without obstetrical service, with school of nursing (5); hospitals without obstetrical service, without school of nursing (7). Cost components are uniformly calculated for each hospital and apply across the four hospital categories, except where a hospital does not maintain a facility. For example, five hospitals are without obstetrical service. "Delivery room," therefore, is not a cost component of the unit cost for these hospitals.

The components for the per diem cost at voluntary hospitals are:

Routine services

Administration and general
Nutrition service: food, other expenses
Operation and maintenance of plant
Laundry and linen service
Housekeeping
Nursing care (excluding training school)
Medical and surgical
Pharmacy
Medical records
Social service
Other

Auxiliary services

Operating rooms
Delivery rooms
X-ray and X-ray therapy
Laboratory
Physical therapy
Electrocardiography
Blood and blood bank
Supplies and drugs sold
Other

Other expenses

Interns and residents
Nurses' training school
Extraordinary repairs and replacements

The 1962 average per diem costs for a general ward patient at the New York Hospital and Mount Sinai Hospital specifically, and for all general voluntary hospitals as an aggregate, were the unit costs employed in this study. The range among the 53 institutions had a low of $24.08 and a high of $51.42. The average cost for all the hospitals was $37.26.

Out-patient Departments: costs per visit. The average cost per OPD visit during the year 1962 at 46 United Hospital Fund member general hospitals was made available to the Project. The unit cost components uniformly apply to all institutions, except where a hospital does not maintain a specific facility, for example, a nurses' training school.

The cost components are:

Routine services

DIRECT EXPENSES
  Salaries and wages
  Supplies and other expenses

ALLOCATED COSTS
  Employees welfare expense
  Administration and general
  Nutrition service
  Operation and maintenance of plant
  Laundry and linen service
  Housekeeping
  Maintenance of personnel
  Nursing care (excluding training school)
  Medical and surgical expenses
  Pharmacy
  Medical records
  Social service
  Other routine service costs

Auxiliary services

  Operating rooms
  X-ray and X-ray therapy
  Supplies and drugs sold
  Other auxiliary services

Other expenses

  Nurses' training school
  Extraordinary repairs and replacements

A unit cost calculated specifically for the New York Hospital and one for Mount Sinai were applied to the utilization of these two hospitals reported by the Project population. For all other voluntary hospital utilization, the average cost for all voluntary general hospitals taken as an aggregate was the unit employed. The per visit costs ranged from $7.02 to $15.24. The average for all 46 hospitals was $9.46.

Department of Health Clinics

Unit costs for four types of Department of Health clinics were calculated specifically for the New York Hospital–Cornell Project cost study by the office of the administrative assistant commissioner.

The type of clinic and the unit cost for each are as follows:

Well-baby clinic—child health stations	$3.74 per visit
Social hygiene clinics	7.52
Chest clinic	9.89
Dental clinic	7.83

Costs for the first three clinics listed were derived from the total expenditures for all facilities in the three categories for the calendar year 1963 and the total number of visits made to each during the same period. The dental visit cost was similarly derived, but it represents cost for the calendar year 1964. The cost components include: personnel (doctor sessions, nursing hours, public health assistants and clerks); general medical supplies; allocated expenses (district and bureau management); overhead, rent, and maintenance.

It was stated that an estimate of $7.00 per visit for all other major services provided by the Department of Health (where "major service" is defined as those facilities utilized by many thousands of patients annually) is a realistic unit cost. Visits to Department of Health cancer detection clinics, because of the comprehensive examination entailed and the few patients serviced, have a considerably greater cost per visit than eye clinics, for example, where examination costs are much less.

Department of Welfare Clinics

The unit cost for a visit to the Department of Welfare eye and dental clinics was calculated by the Project cost staff from information supplied by the office of the assistant to the commissioner. The total expenditure for the Department of Welfare's three eye clinics and four dental clinics and the total number of visits to each for the calendar years 1962 and 1963 were given to the Project. The cost components include: administration; maintenance, laundry, cleaning; professional care; rent and taxes; supplies; dentures and eyeglasses.

State Mental Hospitals and Aftercare Clinics

The per diem cost for state mental hospitals was supplied by the office of the assistant commissioner, State Department of Mental Hygiene. The figures include unit costs for six specific institutions and an average unit cost for all state hospitals for three fiscal years: 1961–62, 1962–63, 1963–64, each beginning with April 1. The 1962–63 average per diem cost for all state hospitals is $6.39. The range in per diem costs for the five hospitals most used by Project patients is: $5.11 to $7.48 for fiscal 1962–63.

Aftercare clinic costs differ in two ways from the costs used in this portion of the study. Per visit costs could not be secured; the expenditure, therefore, is expressed as an average annual cost per patient utilizing aftercare services. And, the expenditure represents reimbursement rather than actual cost to the facility.

The information upon which this calculation is based was supplied by the director of aftercare services in the city of New York. A study conducted between 1959–1961 set the cost of maintaining one patient in aftercare at 10 per cent of the annual reimbursement rate for an institutionalized patient. The fixed annual reimbursement rate was then $2,000. Although reimbursement to state hospitals had increased, the rate reimbursed to aftercare has remained the same. As such, an average annual figure of $200.00 will be used for every patient reporting aftercare utilization.

City Hospitals and Chronic Care Hospitals

Unit cost data relating to the per diem and per visit cost to the institution for city hospitals was made available to the Project cost study by the administrator of the Department of Hospitals. The figures are based on the total expenditure of the Department of Hospitals for the calendar year 1962 and the total in-patient days and OPD visits for the same period.

Per Diem Costs. The average daily costs for general hospitals were derived from the average per diem costs at the 15 general city hospitals. The range depicted was from $30.02 to $49.57. The mean was $38.88; this is the figure used for the "Other city hospitals" category. The additional unit costs employed were those that represent the specific per diem costs at Bellevue and Metropolitan Hospitals.

The figure employed for chronic care hospitals by the cost study was derived from the three city chronic disease hospitals. Per diem costs ranged from $16.73 to $31.97. The mean, $21.87, was applied to all chronic care hospital utilization.

OPD - Per Visit Costs. The fifteen general city hospitals' per visit costs range from $3.92 to $16.18, with a mean of $6.94. This average per visit cost was used for all city hospital OPD utilization, except for that occurring at Bellevue and Metropolitan hospitals. The specific per visit costs for these two institutions was applied to the utilization of their facilities.

Fourteen city hospitals provided the per visit costs for emergency room utilization. These averaged $8.27 per visit and ranged from $3.89 to $13.88. The mean figure was applied to all emergency room utilization, with no one hospital's unit cost separately designated.

According to staff of the United Hospital Fund, the accounting method employed in deriving unit costs for city hospitals is similar to that employed by the UHF. The allocation of general expenses between the in-service and the OPD may differ somewhat from the procedure employed by the UHF, but the overall effect is a slight understatement of unit costs at the city facilities. The components include institutional and divisional expenditures for administration, professional and all other personnel, personnel benefits, rent and maintenance, supplies, and housekeeping and laundry.

Nursing Home Costs

The per diem cost for nursing homes used in the cost study represents reimbursement to the institution by the Department of Welfare. The actual per diem costs to the institution are not available. The information was secured from the supervisor of the Foster Home Program, Bureau of Special Services. The data describes the reimbursement rates from August 1, 1961 to June 30, 1965.

8/1/61 to 3/1/63	$ 8.71
3/1/63 to 4/30/64	10.85
5/1/64 to 6/30/65	11.67

Because the cost study uses 1962 as the cost year, the $8.71 amount is used in nursing home calculations.

Index

ADC, *see* Aid to Dependent Children
Acute hospital care, 136, 150-154, 161-162, 332-333
Acute illness, 6, 90
Aged, 6, 28; decline in symptoms reported by, 40-41
Aid to the Blind, 12, 139, 173
Aid to Dependent Children, 12, 16, 17, 28, 29, 33, 34, 64, 87, 94, 96, 173
Aid to the Disabled, 9, 16, 29, 32, 33, 43, 62, 76, 79, 87, 94, 96, 124, 139, 140, 173, 177, 179
Aid to Families with Dependent Children, 29
Ambulance service, 154, 211
Ambulant medical care, 44, 136, 137-150, 210; costs of, 121-125; sources of, 143-148, 331-332; utilization patterns of Project patients, 148-150
Anemia, 115-116
Annual review, *see* Medical records, review of
Arthur Andersen & Co., 21, 120, 121, 157
Attitude questionnaire, 20, 25, 26, 38, 45-50, 67, 179, 187
Attitudes, 20, 214; to doctors, 48-50, 192-194; to hospitals, 56-57, 198-202; to organization of medical care, 45-48, 190-192; to the Project, 188-190, 195-197; related to mortality study, 177-179; to seeking medical care, 50-56
Audit, medical, 98-100, 110

Baltimore study, 101-104, 209
Barr, Dr. David, 4
Basic scientists, 13
Baumgartner, Leona, 3
"Behavior disorders," defined, 115
Bellevue Hospital, 35, 44, 56, 61, 154, 198, 200, 201, 202, 208, 331, 332; costs at, 159, 161, 162, 168, 169, 337; utilization rates at, 144-149
Blind, 29
Blood test, 18
Board of State Commissioners of Public Charities, 3
Broken appointments, 72-73, 80
Bureau of Nursing, *see* New York City Department of Health
Bus or subway fares, *see* Transportation costs

Capitation payment rate, 12, 17
Case conferences, 87
Chart review, *see* Medical records, review of

Childbirth, 151. *See also* Perinatal care study
Children on welfare, study of, 14, 109-110
Children seen in Project, demographic characteristics of, 108-110
Chronic disease, 3, 6
Chronic institutional care, 136, 154-156, 161-162, 212, 332, 337
Class, in patient-physician relationship, 50
Clerical personnel, 71, 74, 207
Clinic care, preference for, 190-192
Clinic consultations and referrals, 76-78, 79, 210
"Clinic shopper," 7, 150
"Clinical activity status," 83-85
Clinical evaluation, 94-119; methods of, 96-98, 110
Clinical follow-up, *see* Follow-up
Clinical investigation, 13
Clinical liaison, 11
Clinical practice, innovations in, 86
Clinical records, *see* Medical records
Clinical service, communication for, 73
Clinical staff, 70-71
Clinical work-up, 71
Clinicians, 13, 14
Clinics: attitudes to, 44, 45-48, 190-192; costs of care, 158-161; for Project patients, 10, 14, 70-85, 207; for welfare clients in New York City, 8-9, 206; utilization of, 143-150
Commonwealth Fund of New York, 4
Continuity of medical care, 17, 47-48, 92, 129, 163, 191-192, 205, 206, 207, 214
Coordination of medical care, 3, 5-6, 7, 11, 25, 44, 91, 92, 129, 148, 154, 162-163, 165, 192, 205, 207, 210, 213, 215
Cornell Pay Clinic, *see* New York Hospital-Cornell Medical Center
Cornell University Medical College, 3
Costs, 8, 212-213, 334-337; administrative, 163-164; chronic institution, 161-162; general hospital, 161-162; out-patient, 158-161; total estimated, 164-165
Costs, at New York Hospital, 21; in-patient, 125-129; out-patient, 121-125; Project staff, 129-132, 163
Custodial care patients, 89

DRAT, *see* Daily Record of Action Taken
Daily Record of Action Taken (DRAT), 18
Dental care, 9, 10, 91
Dental clinics, 9, 78
Department of Health, *see* New York City Department of Health